ESSENTIALS OF NURSING MANAGEMENT

Quality Assurance

For Nurses and Other Members of the
Health Care Team

Second Edition

Diana Sale

MACMILLAN

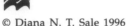

First edition 1990
Reprinted five times
Second edition 1996

Published by
MACMILLAN PRESS LTD
Houndmills, Basingstoke, Hampshire RG21 6XS
and London
Companies and representatives
throughout the world

ISBN 0–333–66917–7

A catalogue record for this book is available
from the British Library.

This book is printed on paper suitable for recycling and
made from fully managed and sustained forest sources.

10 9 8 7 6 5 4 3 2 1
05 04 03 02 01 00 99 98 97 96

Printed in Great Britain by
Antony Rowe Ltd
Chippenham, Wiltshire

This book is dedicated to the memory of my father

Michael Tuke-Hastings
(1920–93)

Contents

Contents

Acknowledgements

I should like to thank the following people who kindly gave me permission to reproduce some of their work in the first edition of this book and which has subsequently been used again in this edition; Dr Alison Kitson (The Royal College of Nursing) and Helen Kendall, Quality Assurance and Standards, Newcastle upon Tyne Polytechnic Products Ltd, for 'Monitor'.

I should also like to thank the new contributors to the second edition of this book. First, Leeds Healthcare for allowing me to use the clinical protocol developed by representatives of St James' Hospital Leeds and myself, and finally Denise Holden of the Dorset Health Commission for the chapter on 'Developing the Commissioning Function of Health Authorities'.

DIANA SALE

Preface

This is the second edition of the book *Quality Assurance* which was first published in 1990. The first edition was intended for nursing staff who were interested in learning more about Quality Assurance and wanted to set up Quality Assurance projects of their own. This book, the second edition, is intended primarily for nurses but I hope that it will also be of interest to other members of the health care team.

Everyone has a part to play in the delivery of high quality care and as we work as multidisciplinary team we should also develop approaches to Quality Assurance as a team. Care of high quality cannot be maintained if members of the same team are working to variable standards. There needs to be an agreed level to which everyone aspires to ensure that patients or clients receive both care and a service of a level that is of good quality.

In order to understand Quality Assurance it is important to have some insight into the background of the subject, which is included in Chapter 1. This chapter has been brought up to date and includes developments and events that have occurred since 1990.

Chapter 2 looks at Total Quality Management (TQM), which is a method of managing quality issues throughout every aspect of an organisation. TQM has been applied all over the world in manufacturing and service industries and with some success in the health care setting. On the one hand it is a 'tool kit' which contains the methods, tools and structure, and on the other hand it is a successful approach to cultural change which promotes a system of continuous quality improvement.

Chapters 3 and 4 set out some of the approaches by which to measure the quality of service and care received by patients or clients and their families or friends. This includes the setting and monitoring of standards and clinical audit.

Chapter 3, on standards, has been changed since the last edition to reflect a simpler and more dynamic approach to setting and, in particular, the monitoring of standards. This approach is based on personal experience and working with a variety of groups since the publication of the first edition of this book.

My work as a management consultant takes me all over the United Kingdom to Acute Hospitals and Community and Mental Health Trusts and I have discovered there is a large variation on the progress made in the area of setting and monitoring of standards. Some staff have done a great deal of very good work on standards while others have done very little. Some are just beginning to think about setting and monitoring standards using a structured approach. Then there are those who say that they have set their standards and hand me a large, dusty tome, written by a committee in 1990. The standards bear no relation to current clinical practice, are not owned or even acknowledged by the staff and have never been monitored. Chapter 3 describes an approach that results in standards that may be seen in everyday practice, that are monitored all the time, based on sound research, valued and owned by the staff and result in good quality care for the patient.

Chapter 4, on clinical audit, is a new addition to the book and sets out one approach to setting up and carrying out an audit. This is a fairly detailed step-by-step guide to audit and is intended for a multidisciplinary approach to audit.

The chapter on clinical protocols (Chapter 5) derives from work undertaken on behalf of Price Waterhouse with St James' Hospital in Leeds, with the kind permission of Leeds Healthcare. This particular approach is a combination of a patient tracking system, anticipated recovery pathways, standards, outcome and workload. The work involved the whole team caring for a patient undergoing a single, first-time hip replacement and tracks the patient's progress from the point of GP referral to discharge.

Chapter 6 looks at the role of the purchaser in Quality Assurance and in particular the monitoring of provider units. This chapter includes a contribution from the Dorset Health

Commission which looks at developing the commission function of Health Authorities.

In each chapter there are exercises to help the readers to put into practice what has been read and to decide whether or not this particular approach is suitable, as a method of Quality Assurance, for the area in which they are working.

This book is intended as a simple, practical guide to Quality Assurance to help staff with the implementation and running of Quality Assurance initiatives.

DIANA SALE

Chapter 1   An Introduction to Quality Assurance

Background

The earliest studies of quality assurance were probably undertaken by the Romans, who must have reported on the efficiency
of their military hospitals. It is also possible that the monks
gave an account of their work in caring for the sick. Probably
the first documented evidence of the evaluation of nursing
care dates back to the eighteenth century, when John Howard
and Elizabeth Fry described the quality of patient care in the
hospitals that they visited.

In the 1850s, Florence Nightingale[1,2] evaluated the care delivered to the sick. She kept notes on her observations and
used the information to establish the level of care being provided and to improve care in areas that were below standard.
During the American Civil War, Louisa M. Alcott[3] wrote about
the quality of nursing care in *Hospital Sketches*, which was
published in 1863. In this publication, she described the con-
trast between the chaos of the 'Hurly-Burly House' and that
of the organised and compassionate care at the Armoury Hospital. At the beginning of this century, between 1920 and 1940,
Isabel Stewart[4] looked at ways of measuring the quality of
nursing care and the effective use of resources. The theory
that quality care is cost effective is still relevant today. She
developed an eight-point list known as Stewart Standards, using
professional opinion rather than a rating scale. The eight-point
list included:

- safety
- therapeutic effect

1

- comfort and general happiness of the patient
- economy of time
- economy of energy and effort
- economy of material and costs
- finished workmanship
- simplicity and adaptability.

In 1936 a book was written by Miss G. B. Carter and Dr H. Balme[5] on the importance of evaluating care. They recommended that a multidisciplinary team, consisting of the ward sister, the doctor and the administrator, should discuss the progress and evaluate the care of all patients, by reviewing the medical and nursing record, at the end of the month. This practice is still in use today when the multidisciplinary team hold a case conference or unit meeting. These meetings are more likely to take place on a weekly basis, when the patients currently being cared for are reviewed and their care evaluated. Discussion is often about the effect of care or treatment, what was effective and what could have been improved.

In the USA in 1958 insurance companies sought to find a standard for assessing quality of care against staffing. As a result, a method was developed by Dr Faye Abdellah[6] that matched staffing levels to the measurement of quality of care in a large hospital. She chose to measure the level of dissatisfaction observed by patients, nurses and other individuals. Over a period of time, she established fifty of the most common causes for dissatisfaction and developed a weighting value for each one. The area of dissatisfaction was rated from five to zero; so, for example, an unconscious patient who was left unattended – and therefore at risk – would have scored five whereas a minor dissatisfaction would have scored zero. The scores were then totalled: a high score indicated poor nursing, whereas a zero score meant that the ward was excellent. Measuring what goes wrong is rather a negative way of evaluating a ward, as it does not measure the positive qualities. This method did not establish that the staffing levels equated with quality of care; in fact, it proved that there was little correlation between the number of staff members and the quality of care. From your own experience, I am sure that you will have observed that having more nurses on a ward does not necessarily mean that patients receive a better standard of care. However, what is important is to note that this system did not offer solutions to resolve dissatisfaction and improve the quality of care.

In the 1950s Frances Reiter[7] developed a system based on the classification of patients into three categories. This classification looked at the way in which nurses plan to work with patients:

- Type 1 was *professional*, where the nurse worked with the patient as in rehabilitation.
- Type 2 was *curative*, where the nurse 'did things' for the patient, such as dressing, treatments and specific tasks.
- Type 3 was *elementary*, *custodial* or *palliative* care; that is, nursing care given to a comatosed or unresponsive patient.

Reiter then developed a series of questions to assess the effectiveness of each type. Her work was published in 1963 and led to a study of communications as a focal point of quality in nursing, which is something that we recognise as essential today.

Since then, nurses all over the world have evaluated the care given to their patients to a greater or lesser degree. In Europe it is really only since 1960 that the evaluation of nursing care has become structured and resulted in systematic studies.

In the 1960s British nursing underwent enormous change with the introduction of the recommendations of the Salmon Report. With the implementation of this Report came the introduction of industrial management techniques and the idea of improving efficiency and saving money in the National Health Service.

In the 1970s accountability and cost effectiveness in the delivery of health care became a major issue and led to the development of systems to help nurses determine the quality of their practice. The 'Nursing Process' from the USA was also introduced in the 1970s and has been adapted and implemented, to a greater or lesser extent, throughout the UK.

In 1974 the government reorganised the National Health Service and set up Area Health Authorities.[8] These were abolished in 1982 with the creation of District Health Authorities, each with its own Community Health Council.[9]

All this change and development led to increased accountability for the quality of the service. In 1974 the Government also set up 'The Office of the Health Service Commissioner' to investigate complaints of maladministration.[10,11] This did not include 'clinical judgement' but the Ombudsman was able to comment on the way complaints were handled and the quality of patient care management.

During the 1960s and 1970s investigations were carried out concerning poor practice, particularly in large institutions caring for the mentally ill and mentally handicapped. This led to the formation of the Hospital Advisory Service for mental illness and elderly care groups, and the National Development Team/ Group for the mentally handicapped. Both these bodies are responsible for inspecting clinical areas and establishing the level of clinical practice. They report on good practice and criticise bad practice. Other forms of audit of quality come from the regular inspection of the academic or validating bodies for training: The National Boards for nursing and the Royal Colleges for postgraduate doctors. They both promote good practice and have the ability to withdraw training from authorities if it is found to be unsatisfactory.

There are also government reports that reflect quality, including the Royal Commission on the National Health Service,[12] the Davies Report and the Griffiths Report.

Since the implementation of the Griffiths Report, the progress on quality assurance programmes throughout the country has accelerated.

Most of the major research on measuring quality of care has been carried out in the USA and Canada. The first studies on quality of nursing care in the USA were developed in the early 1950s, but research on quality evaluation was not undertaken until some years later, when measurement instruments or tools were developed by nurses and researchers from other professional backgrounds. These included the Slater Nursing Competencies Rating Scale,[13] which is a tool designed to measure the nurses' performance, and the Quality Patient Care Scale,[14] which is a tool designed to measure the nursing care received by patients. Nursing Audit by Phaneuf[15] also assesses the quality of patient care by examination of the process of nursing as reflected in the patient's records after discharge.

4

In 1969 Avedis Donabedian[16] divided the evaluation of quality of care into the evaluation of the structure in which care is delivered, the process and the outcome criteria.

In the USA, it was established that audit review alone could not promote an improvement of patient care. Consequently the Joint Commission on Accreditation of Hospitals established standards of nursing care in 1971, giving a more objective and systematic review of patient care and performance. There is also documented evidence of standards setting at the national level in Australia (The Australian Council of Hospital Standards, 1979) and New Zealand (The Joint Commission on Accreditation for Hospitals, 1980).

In the USA, accreditation is linked with funding. If standards fall below predetermined levels, then the hospital organisation is in jeopardy of losing federal or state funding. These hospital accreditation programmes demand evidence that a hospital has some system of quality assurance. Medical audits have developed into medical record audits, which examine in detail the records post-discharge. Today, these systems are often computerised. Some of these hospitals employ a team of people to examine the records and report their findings to a Quality Assurance Committee.

Rush Medicus

The Rush Medicus[17] instrument was developed by the Rush Presbyterian St Luke's Medical Centre and the Medicus Systems Corporation of Chicago from 1972 and was completed in 1975. This system evolved from research in two main areas:

- the development of a 'conceptual framework', stating what is being measured – as this constitutes a patient-centred approach, the nursing process and patient needs were the identified components;
- the identification of criteria for evaluating the quality of care within this framework.

Within the system, there are a series of objectives and sub-objectives, which represent the structure of the nursing process.

At the same time as the development of this system, criteria were developed and tested to measure each of the sub-objectives within the six main objectives. These criteria were written so that a 'yes' or 'no' response indicates the quality of care and, where appropriate, 'not applicable' was applied. Each item was written in such a way as to minimise ambiguity, and to ensure reliable interpretation and response from the observers carrying out the study. If you look through the criteria, you will see that they are relevant to almost any situation of patient care.

The system is computerised and involves a simple dependency rating system, which enables the computer to select 30–50 criteria at random for each patient according to their dependency rating. In order to test the criteria, information is gained by the following methods:

● questioning patients
● questioning nurses
● observing patients
● observing nurses
● observing the patient's environment
● observing the general environment
● examining records
● observer making references.

Rush Medicus developed a method for evaluating the quality of nursing care for medical, surgical and paediatric patients, including the relevant intensive care units. Evaluation is through the production of the two indices. The first is an average score of the quality of patient care and the second is a score for the unit environment. Management Scoring is on a scale of 0–100, where a higher score indicates a better quality of care. The score obtained by the unit is an indication of the quality of care rather than a measure of all aspects of the quality of care.

Monitor

In the UK, Ball *et al.* and Goldstone[18] successfully adapted the Rush Medicus methodology, resulting in the development of the monitoring tool called Monitor. The original version was designed for use on acute surgical and medical wards; however, more recent versions have been developed for use in care of the elderly, wards and district nursing, followed by a version for mental health and paediatric wards in 1987. The midwifery and health visiting versions were published by Leeds Polytechnic in 1989.

Monitor has a patient-orientated approach, and two main concepts: individualised patient care and the patient's needs. Linked with these concepts is the monitoring of the support services who influence the delivery of good standards of patient care.

Monitor is based on a master list of 455 questions about patient care. Only questions 8–150 are directed at the care of any one patient and they are grouped into four sections:

● Assessment and planning
● Physical care
● Non-physical care
● Evaluation.

ASSESSMENT AND PLANNING
● Is there a statement written within 24 hours of admission on the condition of the skin?
● Do the nursing orders or care plan include attention to the patient's need for discharge teaching?

PHYSICAL CARE
● Has the patient received attention to complaints of nausea and vomiting?
● Is adequate equipment for oral hygiene available?

NON-PHYSICAL CARE
● Do the nursing staff call the patient by the name he prefers?
● Are special procedures or studies explained to the patient?

EVALUATION
● Do records document the effect of the administration of 'as required' medication?
● Do records document the patient's response to teaching?

Figure 1 Typical questions representing the different sections of the Monitor patient questionnaire

Monitor follows the structure of the nursing process but the authors state that the clinical area being assessed does not have to be using this approach to patient care in order to use Monitor.

Patients are classified into dependency groups according to the following factors:

● personal care
● feeding
● mobility
● nursing attention (frequency of nursing requirements)
● other (including incontinence, preparation for surgery, severe behavioural problems).

There are four levels of dependence:

● minimal care
● average care
● above average care
● maximum care.

The definitions of dependency are outlined in Figure 2.

There are four different questionnaires, each appropriate to a specific dependency category of patients. The criteria are presented as questions and the information is gained from a variety of sources – by asking the nurse or the patient, consulting records, and observing both the environment and the patient. The questions are answered by a trained assessor with a 'yes', 'no' or 'not applicable' or 'not available'. The scoring system is 1 for 'yes' and 0 for 'no' – the 'not applicable' or 'not available' answers are deleted. The total score is given as the percentage of 'yes' responses obtained. The closer the score is to 100 percent, the better the standard of care being delivered.

CATEGORY I – MINIMAL CARE

Patient is physically capable of caring for himself but requires minimal nursing supervision and may require treatments and/or monitoring (e.g., B.P., T.P.R. clinical observations) by nursing staff.

CATEGORY II – AVERAGE CARE
Patient requires an average or moderate amount of nursing care, including some nursing supervision and help with personal care needs as well as monitoring and treatments. Some examples would include:

- a patient past the acute stage of his disease or surgery
- a 3–4 day post-op cholecystectomy
- a diabetic patient for reassessment
- an independent patient requiring extensive investigative procedure.

CATEGORY III – ABOVE AVERAGE CARE
Patient requires a greater than average amount of nursing care, including nursing supervision, encouragement and almost complete assistance to meet personal care needs. The patient usually requires medical support and sometimes the use of special equipment. Some examples would be:

- a patient after the acute phase of CVA (residual paralysis)
- a first day post-op radical mastectomy or cholecystectomy
- a debilitated, dependent elderly person
- a newly diagnosed diabetic requiring extensive health teaching and support from nursing staff.

CATEGORY IV – MAXIMUM CARE
Patient requires very frequent to continuous nursing care along with close supervision by medical personnel and/or health team members, and/or support from the technical equipment. Some examples would include:
- a quadriplegic in early rehabilitative stages
- a severely burned patient
- a comatose patient.

Figure 2 Definition of categories

From: Ball *et al.*, *Monitor: An Index of the Quality of Nursing Care for Acute Medical and Surgical Wards* (Newcastle-upon-Tyne Polytechnic Products Ltd, 1983)

'In Pursuit of Excellence'

In 1985 the Royal College of Nursing Standards of Care Project was set up with the intention of establishing the academic background to quality of care and to encourage the nursing profession to set and monitor standards.

The Royal College of Nursing published two significant papers, which are essential reading for anyone who is interested in the history of quality assurance; they are 'Standards of Nursing Care' (1980)[19] and 'Towards Standards' (1981).[20] Dr Alison Kitson's work with the RCN led to the active setting and monitoring of standards within the nursing profession, and her published work includes 'Indicators of Quality in Nursing Care – an Alternative Approach' (1986),[21] 'Taking Action' (1986),[22] and 'Rest Assured' (1986).[23]

In 1987 the RCN produced a positive statement on nursing, 'In Pursuit of Excellence'. The steering group which produced this statement set down three main principles: equity, respect for persons, and caring. The group then provided nine statements to enable nurses to move to the provision of a 'quality service' based on core concepts.

Since the publication of the first edition of this book the work in setting and monitoring standards has marched on and is discussed in Chapter 3.

'Working for Patients'

In 1983, when the Griffiths Recommendations and General Management of health care were introduced, quality assurance and the establishment of standards and review mechanisms became the responsibility of all General Managers at Regional, District and Unit level.

In 1985 Alain Enthoven, an American university professor, studied the organisation of the NHS and suggested that it could be improved by the introduction of an 'Internal Market Model'. He envisaged a system that would enable District Managers to use services more efficiently. The system, very briefly, would be that each District would receive, under a formula drawn up by the Resource Allocation Working Party (RAWP), a per capita revenue and capital allowance. The District would be responsible for the provision of comprehensive care for its own resident population, but not for patients from other Districts without current compensation at negotiated prices. The District would buy and sell services to other Districts and the private sector. Alain Enthoven's work was an influence in the thinking behind the National Health Service and Community Care Act 1990.

This 1990 legislation facilitated the development of the process of contracting between the purchaser and the provider units. The provider units in the form of NHS Trusts and Directly Managed Units (DMUs) are responsible for meeting specifications for services as laid down in the contract with the purchaser (commissioner). The purchaser (commissioner) is looking for value for money and quality care from the providers. In Chapter 6 an approach provided by the Dorset Health Commission expands on monitoring the quality of care provided by the provider units.

Medical Audit

As part of the NHS reforms the government facilitated the development of programmes intended to measure and improve the quality of care within the NHS. One particular initiative was the development of medical audit. Over the years there have been studies which audited the quality of medical care, including a survey of general practice by Collings in 1950.[24] Collings established that there was poor quality of care and his survey contributed to the formation in 1952 of the College of General Practitioners, which is now known as the Royal College of General Practitioners. Collings' study observed current practice and found it to be lacking but his findings did not directly change the delivery of care. However, another study, 'The Confidential Enquiry into Maternal Deaths',[25] focused on the reasons for inadequate care and the results led to changes in practice and a reduction in maternal deaths.

In 1967, in the Cogwheel report, audit was described as a

proper function for practising clinicians,[26] but there was still a distinct lack of mechanisms for monitoring the effectiveness of patient care. In the 1970s the General Medical Council was criticised for its inability to stop doctors over-prescribing heroin and other addictive drugs to patients[27] and there were concerns that Britain had not become involved in audit.

In the 1960s a series of events led to a more active approach to audit. There was the UK national quality control scheme for clinical chemistry analyses in hospital laboratories,[28] and the establishment of the Hospital Advisory Service (HAS) in 1969.[29] In 1976 (Lament Report) and again in 1979 (Morrison Report) Royal Commissions stressed the importance of audit. In 1975, the radiologists established a working party on the use of diagnostic radiology[30] and later in 1977 the physicians founded the Medical Service Group.[31] In 1978 the Conference of Senior Hospital Staff passed a resolution on medical audit. The following year in 1979, The Royal Commission on The National Health Service (Morrison Report) emphasised the importance of audit. During the 1980s there was further activity from the Royal College of General Practitioners (1980). In 1984 the government signed a declaration that effective mechanisms for quality of health care would be in place by 1990 (WHO Health Policy, 1984). Again the Royal College of General Practitioners issued a policy statement 'Quality in General Practice' (1985). In 1987 the Royal College of Surgeons declared a requirement that regular audit was necessary for training posts to be recognised.

In 1989 the Royal College of Physicians published a report on Medical Audit and the Department of Health published the White Paper 'Working for Patients'.

The introduction and early progress of medical audit was slow but has gathered speed during the last ten years. Perhaps due to the NHS tradition of professional autonomy, audit has been seen as operating in separate areas, medical audit, clinical audit and nursing audit. During the 1990s there has been an ever increasing number of audits undertaken by professionals either as a uniprofessional group or on a multidisciplinary basis. The principles of audit apply whether undertaken by a group of professionals from the same background or the multidisciplinary team. In Chapter 4 I have

developed the principles of audit and included examples of
audits undertaken by various members of the health care team.

Defining Quality Assurance

There are many definitions of the term 'quality assurance' written by people who have researched the subject thoroughly. A
definition that I feel is both appropriate and easily understood
is that given by Williamson: 'Quality assurance is the measurement of the actual level of the service provided plus the
efforts to modify when necessary the provision of these services in the light of the results of the measurement.'[32] Another definition, according to Schmadl, is as follows: 'The
purpose of quality assurance is to assure the consumer of
nursing of a specified degree of excellence through continuous measurement and evaluation.'[33]

The word 'quality' is defined by the Concise Oxford Dictio-
nary as 'degree of excellence' and the word 'assurance' means
'formal guarantee; positive declaration'. So, from these definitions, 'quality assurance' may be interpreted as a formal guarantee of a degree of excellence. In other words, it assures patients
of an acceptable standard of care.

Levels of Monitoring the Quality of Care

There are various levels at which the monitoring of the quality of patient care may take place. Nationally there are several major programmes which monitor externally the quality
of care in the health service. These include:

- The Audit Commission
- Organisational Audit through the King's Fund Centre
- the application of the International and British Standards
  in Quality Systems (ISO 9000/BS 5750) to health care services
- compliance with the Patient's Charter

Under the NHS Reform Act, a Clinical Standards Advisory

Group, accountable to the Secretary of State, has been established to monitor standards in the NHS. Also, the Audit Commission is empowered to audit the NHS and includes evaluation of aspects of quality of service.

The Audit Commission

The Audit Commission has been responsible for the external audit of the National Health Service in England and Wales since October 1990. The Audit Commission has responsibility for reviewing the financial accounts of all health service bodies and examining the health authorities' use of resources for economy, efficiency and effectiveness.

Some of the most recent studies include:

- *Lying in Wait: The Use of Medical Beds in Acute Hospitals* (1992)
- *The Virtue of Patients: Making Best Use of the Usual Nursing Resources* (1991)
- *Children First* (1993)
- *Seen But Not Heard – Welfare of Children and Young People in the Community* (1994)
- *Purchaser* (1994)
- *A Short Cut to Better Services: Day Surgery in England and Wales* (1990)
- *Value for Money in NHS Sterile Services* (1991)

The aim of the Audit Commission is to help people who work in and manage the NHS to deliver the best possible service within the financial resources determined by government.

Each year the Audit Commission publishes a number of reports on health topics which have been researched at a national level. The Audit Commission then ensures that local audits are carried out on each topic. The national reports are not intended to be comprehensive surveys because most of the detailed information is collected by auditors during the audits that follow the publication of the report. The reports are intended to highlight the national issues established through the study.

The national studies are carried out by a team consisting of professionals relevant to the subject. They involve detailed examination of a number of study sites, with the combination of published research and analysis of national data. The study team is supported by an advisory group consisting of individuals with a close interest in the subject.

The local studies are undertaken by management consultants and the Audit Commission staff. The auditors follow the Audit Commission guidelines, review local policies and procedures, interview staff, observe the particular service, and review activity and staffing data. They also review national guidelines, information, activity and staffing data. At the end of the study a report is written which is discussed with the management team, and an action plan is agreed and drawn up with the main objective – to improve the service for the patient.

King's Fund Organisational Audit

In November 1988 The Quality Assurance programme at the King's Fund Centre organised a conference to consider the development of national standards for the organisation of health care. Six District Health Authorities – Brighton, East Dorset, North Derbyshire, North West Hertfordshire, Nottingham (Queen's Medical Centre) and West Dorset – were selected to participate in the project. In addition, two independent hospitals, the Hospital of St John and St Elizabeth and AMI Chiltern, joined the project. A project steering group looked critically at existing systems for setting and monitoring national standards, principally those models of accreditation used in the USA, Canada and Australia. The group considered the Australian system to be the most appropriate on which to build its own model, with reference to the Canadian system as appropriate. The King's Fund Organisational Audit was established in 1989, with the development of national standards for acute hospitals. By 1994 approximately 150 hospitals had been surveyed by the King's Fund Organisational Audit which was extended into Health Centres and GP practices in 1992, with the Primary Health Care Project, and into community hospitals, with a pilot study in 1994.

Accreditation

Accreditation is a method which is used to address the issues of evaluating the quality of health services provided. It is the 'professional and national recognition reserved for facilities that provide high quality health care. This means that the particular health care facility has voluntarily sought to be measured against high professional standards and is in substantial compliance with them' (Limongelli, 1983).[34]

Accreditation is a system of organisational audit and is made up of three stages:

1. The development of organisational standards which are concerned with the systems and process for the delivery of health care – the standards are developed in consultation with the relevant professional organisations and are revised annually to ensure that they reflect current health care trends;
2. Implementation of standards – the various accreditation agencies provide support material and guidelines on interpretation of standards;
3. Evaluation of compliance with standards by means of a survey, conducted by a team of trained surveyors chosen for their expertise in a specific health care service.

Accreditation differs from both registration and licensing in that it is not a statutory but a voluntary system.[35] At the time of writing (1995) accreditation has not been established in the UK, but it would appear that it is only a matter of time before accreditation is part of our quality assurance programme.

Levels of Evaluation of Quality of Care

There are various levels at which evaluation of the quality of care may take place. It may be at national level – for example, the standards set in the USA by the American Nurses' Association; in Canada by the four Canadian Nurses' Associations (the Canadian Nurses' Association,[36] The College of Nurses of Ontario,[37] the Ordre des Infirmières et Infirmiers du Quebec,[38] and the Manitoba Association of Registered Nurses[39]); and in

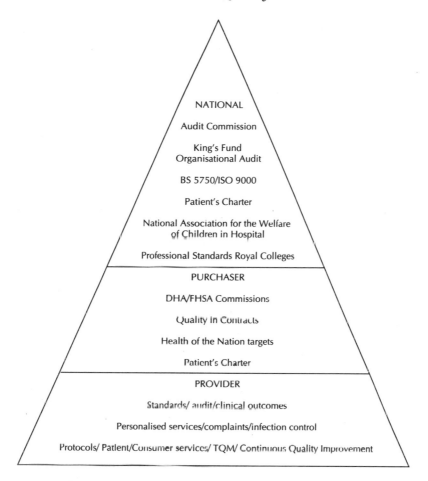

Figure 3 Levels of evaluation of the quality of care

Australia by the Royal Australian Nursing Federation.[40]

In Figure 3, 'Levels of evaluation of the quality of care', the top level may be seen as the 'national level'. At this level there are a variety of organisations in the UK which undertake structured audits of Trusts and other organisations and these include the Audit Commission and the King's Fund Organisational Audit, as mentioned above.

At this level the organisation is measured against pre-set standards or criteria by a team from outside the organisation.

While employed within the NHS, I have been involved in various studies led by an outside auditor. At first it seemed rather threatening as we prepared ourselves for the audit, but as the preparations progressed we began to realise just how much the organisation had achieved over the previous few years. It is very easy to continue to work hard, day by day, to improve the service without taking the opportunity to reflect on what has been achieved. Preparing for an audit, and in particular the King's Fund Organisational Audit, gives staff an opportunity to stand back and reflect on what has been achieved, and by the end of the survey they will have a much clearer picture of how to move forward.

Also at this top level are standards set by the Royal Colleges and the professional organisations such as the Chartered Society of Physiotherapists, the Patient's Charter and British Standard BS 5750 and ISO 9000.

The next level is that of the Purchaser and the areas of Quality Assurance may well be within the contract as indicators of quality or specified standards. The quality issues addressed in the contract may focus on the Health of the Nation targets, the Patient's Charter, or areas of concern identified by the consumer and the Community Health Council. The purchaser will also focus on national issues which have arisen from other studies – for example, skill mix in the Community Nursing Service.

The next and most important level is the clinical area, the wards, departments, unit, clinics, GP practices. Here the quality assurance activities may be varied and numerous. Within the concept of this book, I shall be concentrating on this level, looking at ways of measuring the quality of care in the wards, departments, clinics and the patient's home. Until recently quality assurance has been monitored by groups of professionals, often in isolation from the rest of the caring team. However, this is not true to life, as in the majority of health care settings the patient is cared for by a team of professionals. For example, the patient when admitted for surgery is not cared for exclusively by a surgeon. The nursing staff have a part to play, the anaesthetist is involved, the patient may need the services of the radiologist, the pathologist, the pharmacists, the therapist, the phlebotomist, the ECG technician, the porters, the clerks and many others. By measuring the quality of care delivered by just one group of staff within the team, we are only measuring a small part of the care, and what is not measured is how care delivered by one professional impacts upon the care given by another. There is also an opportunity to be more efficient and effective by discussing who does what, when, how and by identifying the outcome for the patient. And it is important to establish what the organisation as a whole is developing, and what is taking place both at a national and regional level, so that you can be an effective part of the quality assurance programme.

Evaluation of Quality of Care

There are a variety of conceptual models of evaluation that have been published and may be used by anyone, from any background, as a model of evaluation. Norma Lang's model[41] was adapted by the American Nurses' Association and modified by Vail in 1986, when an eighth step was added. Lang's model was also adapted by the Royal Australian Nursing Federation to include eleven steps, as shown in Figure 4. The model can also be adapted as shown in Figure 5, for use by a quality assurance committee, or for the ward sister or charge nurse, head of department, or professionals in their particular clinical area.

Before developing a framework for measuring the quality of care on your ward or clinical area, it is essential to establish what has already been written and researched. A great deal of work has been done and it will help you to select a framework that will suit your needs. There is no need to reinvent the wheel, so a literature search will save you a great deal of time and energy. I hope that within this book there will be enough information to help you with this activity.

The first step of the quality cycle is to get together with colleagues in your clinical area and write a philosophy of care. To do this, you need to discuss your personal beliefs about patient care, the profession's code of conduct, beliefs about the uniqueness of individuals and their human rights, the

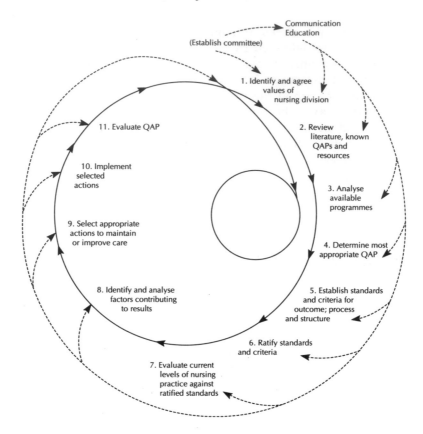

Figure 4 Steps in implementing a quality assurance programme (QAP): Model for quality assurance

From: N. Lang, 'Issues in Quality Assurance in Nursing', *ANA Issues in Evaluative Research* (American Nursing Association, 1976).

philosophy of care of the health district and society's values. This does not have to be a long, detailed account but simply a summary of your beliefs as a caring team of professionals.

The next step is to set some objectives – what you hope to achieve by measuring the quality of care. This should include the measurable effect of care given to patients and the performance of the staff involved in the delivery of patient care.

Before you can measure the quality of care, you must be able to describe what you do. To this end, it is necessary to identify standards and criteria. On reviewing the literature,

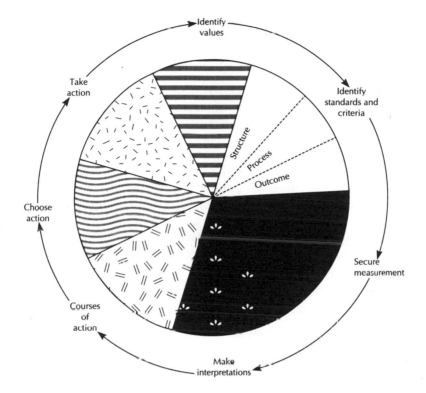

Figure 5 Adapted quality assurance model

you will find that a number of tools have been developed and are in use all over the country. Many approaches are based on criteria and standards, and can be categorised into a structure, process and outcome framework. Some authors of these tools favour the measurement of process while others favour outcome.

To measure the quality of care, the appropriate tool must be selected. The tools are essentially data collection systems using retrospective and concurrent audit; that is, systems for collecting information which, when collated, will give an indication of the quality of patient care for a particular ward or department.

1. Retrospective audit

Retrospective audit involves all assessment mechanisms carried out after the patient has been discharged. These include:

- **closed-chart auditing**, which is the review of the patient records and identification of strengths and deficits of care. This can be achieved by a structured audit of the patient's records;
- **post-care patient interview**, which is carried out when the patient has left the hospital or care has ceased in the home. It involves inviting the patient and/or family members to meet to discuss experiences. This may be unstructured, semi-structured or structured using a checklist or questionnaire.
- **post-care questionnaires**, which should be completed by the patient on discharge. They are usually designed to measure patient satisfaction.

2. Concurrent audit

Concurrent audit involves all assessments performed while the patient is in hospital and receiving care. These include:

- **open-chart auditing**, which is the review of the patient's charts and records against preset criteria. As the patient is still receiving care, this process gives staff immediate feedback;
- **patient interview or observation**, which involves talking to the patient about certain aspects of care, conducting a bedside audit or observing the patient's behaviour to preset criteria;
- **staff interview or observation**, which involves talking to and observing nursing behaviour related to preset criteria;
- **group conferences**, which involve the patient and/or family in joint discussion with staff about the care being received. This leads to problems being discussed and improved plans agreed.

The advantages and disadvantages of these tools will be discussed in the following chapters. Evaluation of the results involves comparing 'what is' with 'what should be' and then identifying what needs to be done to achieve quality care.

'Taking action' is achieved by developing a plan to ensure that care is given according to the agreed standard. If this last vital step is not taken, then there has been little point in the exercise, and there will be no improvement of patient care. Where standards are found to be low, or where there is poor quality of care, action must be planned and taken to change practice, and the cycle starts again.

Exercise 1

In order to take the first step of this cycle, you could start by
discussing and then writing a philosophy and objectives for the
patients in your clinical area. To help with this exercise, consider the
following points.

- Establish if the Trust or organisation that you work for has a
  philosophy of care and objectives. Check with your manager or
  look through the Business Plan or the Quality Assurance Plan.
- If there is a statement of philosophy and objectives, then check
  that it can be used as a guide to plan, implement and evaluate all
  aspects of the service.
- Then use it to develop a philosophy and objectives for the patients
  in your clinical area.

If there is no statement of philosophy and consequent objectives,
then the structure proposed, and the advice given by Marjorie Moore
Cantor,[42] may be helpful. It is important to note that she stated very
clearly that there was no justification in having a philosophy that
could not be used to support and develop practice and improve
patient care. She also denounced the use of very broad abstract terms
and concepts wrapped up in jargon. A philosophy needs to be
written so that it can be easily understood by all concerned, and is
not open to misinterpretation. The structure or framework has three
parts:

- *The purpose* This statement describes the reason for being – the
  why of the service. It tries to answer the question: 'What is the
  purpose of patient care?'
- *The philosophy* This is a statement of belief that identifies how
  the purpose should be achieved and provides an explanation of
  how it is derived. The purpose and philosophy form the basis of
  policies and practice and objectives. Some areas to consider when
  developing a philosophy of care are: the nature of health and ill
  health; people's relationships to health and ill health; the role of
  the professional in health and ill health; people's needs,
  professional's needs and inter-professional collaboration.
- *The objectives* These must contain criteria, which are items or
  variables that are measurable, in order to evaluate the degree to
  which the purpose is achieved. Many of the statements made in
  the philosophy will translate into objectives. There is plenty of
  literature on the subject, so ask the library to do a literature
  search for you. Outside the district or organisation, you could
  contact the Royal Colleges, the King's Fund, professional
  organisations.

When you have written your philosophy and objectives, you need to
check the following:

➤

- Do they reflect the beliefs and objectives of all the staff involved in patient care?
- Does your philosophy reflect that of the Trust or organisation?
- Do the objectives reflect the philosophy of the Trust or organisation?
- Do the philosophy and objectives reflect the patient's and his/her family's needs?
- Have the philosophy and the objectives been acknowledged by other members of the caring team?
- Have managers acknowledged the philosophy and objectives?

References

1. Nightingale, F., *Notes on Matters Affecting the Health, Efficiency and Hospital Administration of the British Army* (Garrison, 1858).
2. Nightingale, F., Address from Florence Nightingale to the probationer nurses in the Nightingale Fund School at St Thomas's Hospital who were formerly trained there. Printed for private use 23 July 1874 (Nutting Collection, Teachers College, Columbia University).
3. Alcott, L. M., *Hospital Sketches*. ed. Bessie Z. Jones (Cambridge: The Belknap Press of Harvard University Press, 1960).
4. Stewart, I., 'Possibilities of Standardisation of Nursing Techniques', *Modern Hospital* (1919) **12**(6), 451–4.
5. Carter, G. B. and H. Balme, *Importance of Evaluating Care* (1936).
6. Abdellah, F., *Effects of Nursing Staffing on Satisfactions with Nursing Care* (American Hospital Association Monograph, 1958).
7. Reiter, F. and M. Kakosh, *Quality of Nursing Care: A Report of a Field Study to Establish Criteria 1950–1953* (New York Graduate School of Nursing, New York Medical College, 1963).
8. DHSS, The National Health Service Reorganisation Act, 1973 (London: HMSO, 1973).
9. DHSS, The *NHS (Constitution of District Health Authorities)* (London: HMSO, 1981).
10. DHSS, *NHS Management Enquiry* (London: DHSS, 1983).
11. DHSS, *Report of the Committee on Hospital Complaints Procedure* (London: HMSO, 1985).
12. DHSS, *Royal Commission on the National Health Service* (C 7615) London: DHSS, 1979).
13. Wandelt, M. A. and S. D. Stewart, *Slater Nursing Competencies Rating Scale* (Detroit: Appleton–Century–Crofts, 1975).
14. Wandelt, M. A. and J. W. Ager, *Quality Patient Care Scale* (New York: Appleton–Century–Crofts, 1974).

15. Phaneuf, M., *The Nursing Audit* (Detroit: Appleton–Century–Crofts, 1972).
16. Donabedian, A., 'Medical Care Appraisal – Quality and Utilization' in *Guide to Medical Care Administration*, vol. 11 (New York: American Public Health Association, 1969).
17. Hegyvary, S. T. and R. K. D. Hausman, 'Monitoring Nursing Care Quality', *Journal of Nursing Administration* (1975) **15**(55), 17–26.
18. Goldstone, L. and J. Ball, 'The Quality of Nursing Services', *Nursing Times* (1984) **29**(8), 56–9.
19. Royal College of Nursing, *Standards of Nursing Care* (London, 1980).
20. Royal College of Nursing, *Towards Standards* (London, 1981).
21. Kitson, A., 'Indicators of Quality in Nursing Care – An Alternative Approach', *Journal of Advanced Nursing* (1986) **11**(2), 133–44.
22. Kitson, A., 'Taking Action', *Nursing Times* (1986) **3**, 52–4.
23. Kitson, A. and H. Kendall, 'Rest Assured', *Nursing Times* (1986) **27**, 28–31.
24. Collings, J. S., 'General Practice in England Today: A RECONNAISSANCE', *Lancet* (1950), 535–8?.
25. Godber, G., 'The Confidential Enquiry into Maternal Deaths', in G. McLachlan (ed.) *A Question of Quality* (London: Oxford University Press, 1976) 24–33.
26. Williamson, J. D., 'Quality Control, medical audit and the general practioner', *Journal of the Royal College of General Practitioners* (1973) **23**, 697–706.
27. Dollery, C. T., 'The quality of health care', in G. McLachlan (ed.) *Challenge for change* (London: Oxford University Press, 1971).
28. Whitehead, T., 'Surveying the performance of pathological laboratories', in G. McLachlan (ed). *A Question of Quality* (London: Oxford University Press 1976) 97–117.
29. Baker, A., 'The Hospital Advisory Service', in G. McLachlan (ed.) *A Question of Quality* (London: Oxford University Press, 1976) 203–16.
30. Roberts, C. J., 'Annotation: towards the more effective use of diagnostic radiology: a review of the work of the Royal College of Radiologists' working party on the more effective use of diagnostic radiology, 1976–1988', *Clinical Radiology* (1988) **39**, 3–6.
31. Clarke, C. and A. G. W. Whitehead, 'The collaboration of the Medical Services Group to the Royal College of Physicians to improvement in care', in G. McLachlan (ed.) *Reviewing Practice in Medical Care: Steps to Quality Assurance* (London: Nuffield Provincial Hospital Trust, 1981) 33–40.
32. Williamson, J. W., 'Formulating Priorities for Quality Assurance Activity: Description of Method and its Application', *Journal of the American Medical Association* (1978) **239**, 631–7.
33. Schmadl, J. C., 'Quality Assurance: Examination of the Concept', *Nursing Outlook* (1979) **27**(7), 462–5.

34. Limongelli, F., 'Accreditation: new standards published', *Dimensions in Health Services* (1983) **60**, 18–19.
35. Higgins, J., 'A Consultation on the Accreditation of Residential Care Homes, Nursing Homes and Mental Nursing Homes: a report of, and commentary upon, a conference held at the King's Fund Centre on 25 January 1985', Project Paper no. 56.
36. Canadian Nurses' Association, 'Development of a Definition of Nursing Practice', *The Canadian Nurse* (1980) **76**(5), 11–15.
37. College of Nurses of Ontario, 'The Standards and Levels of Nursing Practice Including the Assumptive Base (A discussion paper)' (1985).
38. Ordre des Infirmières et Infirmiers du Quebec, 'Standards and Criteria of Competence for Nurses', extracts from *Education of the Professional Competence of the Nurse in Quebec* (Ordres des Infirmières et Infirmiers du Quebec, 1985).
39. Manitoba Association of Registered Nurses, 'Standards of Nursing Care' (Manitoba: MARN, 1981).
40. Royal Australian Nursing Federation, *Standards for Nursing Practice* (Melbourne: Royal Australian Nursing Federation, 1983).
41. Lang, N., 'Issues in Quality Assurance in Nursing', *ANA Issues in Evaluative Research* (American Nursing Association, 1976).
42. Cantor, M. M., 'Philosophy, Purpose and Objectives: Why Do We Have Them?, *The Journal of Nursing Administration* (1971) **5**(6), 9–14.

Further Reading

Fawcett, R., 'Measurement of Care Quality', *Nursing Mirror* (1985) **160**(2), 29–31.

Jelinek, R. C. et al., *A Methodology for Monitoring Quality of Nursing Care* (Bethesda, Md.: US Department for Education, Health and Welfare publ. no. (HRA) 76–25, 1976).

Jelinek, R. C., et al., *Monitoring Quality of Nursing Care, Part 2, Assessment and Study of Correlates* (Bethesda, Md.: US Department of Education, Health and Welfare publ. no (HRA) 76–7, 1976).

Jelinek, R. C. et al., *Monitoring Quality of Nursing Care Part 3, Professional Review for Nursing: An Empirical Investigation* (Bethesda, Md,: US Department of Education, Health and Welfare publ. no. (HRA) 77–70, 1977).

Illsley, V. A. and L. A. Goldstone, *Guide to Monitor* (Newcastle-upon-Tyne Polytechnic Products Ltd, 1986).

McCall, J., 'Monitor Evaluated', *Senior Nurse* (1988) **8**(5), 8–9.

Whelan, J., 'Using Monitor – Observer Bias', *Senior Nurse* (1987) **7**(6), 8–10.

Chapter 2   Total Quality Management

Background

Total Quality Management (TQM) was developed in the USA by W. E. Deming[1] and J. M. Juran[2] as a business philosophy to improve market performance. Their philosophy was welcomed and implemented in Japan in the 1980s. TQM was widely practised by Japanese businesses and is the foundation of the country's economic dominance today. Japanese businesses reviewed the way that they operated and managed to achieve the competitive edge based on producing better goods at better prices than their competitors in the West.

This same philosophy may be used to improve the quality of service in the health service by looking critically at what is really needed to produce quality goods or, in this case, service. The factory needs to work well as a team and so does the hospital. If there are delays or defects in the service then the customer will be dissatisfied with the service.

In 1990 the Department of Health selected 23 demonstration sites to introduce a system of a managed approach to quality, or TQM. The sites ranged from departments within units, to hospitals, to entire districts and they were part funded by the Department of Health. Some common themes which help define a total quality NHS emerged from the demonstration sites and included[3]:

- actively seeking patients' views and building organisations around their needs
- encouraging staff to respond positively to patients' needs and suggestions

- top management and professional commitment to quality
- creating a culture which encourages wide involvement and devolves responsibility to front-line staff
- systematic training for staff to equip them with the skills they need to participate in change
- effective communications
- continuous improvement based on systematic measurement.

Quality has always been an essential aspect of the delivery of professional care but TQM moves the focus from quality practised within the professions to the organisation as a whole. The key principles and strategies of TQM include customer focus, teamwork, breaking down professional barriers and better management of resources.

Total Quality Management is a method of managing quality issues throughout every aspect of an organisation, ensuring that everyone gets it right, first time, every time. It is also about developing a culture where all the staff strive to get it right, first time, every time and do not pass on errors and mistakes to someone else in the organisation.

TQM has been applied all over the world in manufacturing and service industries. TQM involves the whole organisation becoming organised as far as quality is concerned and that means everyone in every department.

Mistakes, errors and poor practice may be serious in a manufacturing organisation but in the health care setting they can be devastating. The cost of poor quality care is so much greater than the cost of good quality care.

For example, a patient is admitted for a hip replacement operation, the patient is well prepared for surgery, the surgical intervention is excellent and the patient returns to the ward. So far so good, but on the ward there is a problem, the nurses are short of staff due to sickness and there is no money in the budget to replace the total staffing numbers with bank or agency staff. So the nursing team is reduced to two members of staff for 28 patients, of whom 10 have returned from theatre that day.

Because of this our patient is still lying on a theatre canvas, which is rough to the skin, and the skin is already red. Our patient is not able to move herself around the bed and inevitably develops a pressure sore, which will take time to heal.

This will slow down the rehabilitation process and increase the length of stay, which will cost more – and this takes no account of the unnecessary pain, discomfort and inconvenience to the patient. There is also, of course, a 'knock on' effect on the waiting list, which will leave another patient in pain for longer than anticipated.

This is just one example of how poor quality of care costs money, but there are other examples which include delay in care being delivered; the unnecessary testing and treatment of patients; the necessity to repeat care to rectify errors; poor patient care and service, with non-compliance to explicit and implicit standards; the result of errors and misjudgements leading to unnecessary and expensive litigation; the recall of patients for repeat tests and treatments that perhaps were not done correctly the first time.

There are numerous examples, and I am sure that you can cite several from your own working environment.

Concepts

The concepts of TQM are fairly simple. Any organisation requires 'processes' for ensuring that the service it provides is needed by the consumer and is of an acceptable standard. In a Department of Trade and Industry publication in 1989 John Oakland outlined the TQM processes as follows. The organisation should:

- focus on the needs and expectations of its market and its consumers
- achieve top quality performance in all areas of its activity (product, service and internal processes)
- instal and operate procedures, simple and complex, necessary for the achievement of top quality performance
- critically and continuously examine processes to reduce and remove non-productive activities, inefficiencies and waste
- develop and monitor measures of performance, set standards against which this performance is measured and set required improvements.

- understand and develop an effective communication strategy
- develop a non-hierarchical team approach to problem-solving and delegating responsibility for change
- develop good procedures for communication and feedback to staff at any level of good work
- continuously review the above processes to develop a culture for never-ending improvement.

(Source: John Oakland, 1989, Department of Trade and Industry)

In the business world companies have constantly to address issues of quality to ensure that they are not overtaken by their competitors: the consumer demands a high quality product or service. Since the NHS reforms this is also becoming the case in the Health Service.

Patient awareness and expectations have been raised by the Patient's Charter. GPs will refer patients to the service that is responsive, effective and efficient and not to the hospital or service where there are waiting lists or a history of poor quality.

TQM can enable a Trust to meet patients' needs through an organised approach to monitoring and enhancing the quality of care or service delivered by all the staff. In order to do this there must be a commitment by all the staff to improve the quality of service to patients and their families.

In the past within the Health Service there has tended to be a 'top down' approach to quality assurance, people with the responsibility for quality, developing standards and distributing them to wards and departments for 'comments' prior to the standards being implemented. TQM is about the development of a culture in which all staff are involved in ways of improving care and are supported by a management system with the same commitment to quality improvement.

TQM is about meeting and *exceeding* the consumers' requirements. These may be the requirements of the GPs, patients and patients' families. To do this there must be ways of establishing what the patients or GPs require of the service and developing ways of responding to this need, by understanding not only the external customer but also the internal staff requirements.

Another key aspect of this approach is the monitoring of the standard of the service by constant review of the key elements. It is necessary to ensure that standards set are indeed true standards that are explicit, measurable, a true reflection of quality and include patients and relatives using the service. The whole organisation needs to be clear about the need for compliance with these standards and the implications of non-compliance.

Perhaps the key issue of all those mentioned is the issue of ownership and commitment to quality of care and service by all staff, at all levels of the organisation. Historically staff within the health service have been committed to delivering quality care and have worked hard to improve the care they give and the service they deliver. The main difference is that instead of having pockets of enthusiasm within the organisation, the whole organisation is part of a structured system of quality that is managed systematically. TQM should encourage every member of staff to be an active cog in the quality wheel, to be loyal to the hospital and department and support staff to deliver higher quality and cost effective care and services.

In 1989 DHAs were instructed, through paper EL(89)M3117, to ensure that their units developed systematic and continuing review of quality, using a format and contents determined locally but consistent with national and regional policies. They were instructed to monitor all aspects of quality of patient care and service, including outcome. The specific areas included:

- medical and clinical audit
- reducing waiting times (outpatient and inpatient)
- specification of quality elements to contracts
- measurable criteria or standards of care and service
- improved appointment systems
- information to patients
- reception and public area arrangements
- customer feedback on strategies
- improved environments (for example, in Accident & Emergency).

Approach

The TQM approach is about putting the needs of patients at the centre of every activity at all levels of the organisation with the support and involvement of management, as demonstrated in Figure 6.

Exercise 2

Either on your own or in a group develop a diagram similar to Figure 6 and complete it for your own organisation. Establish what quality initiatives are being undertaking, what support systems there are in the organisation and establish if the organisation that you work in is one which uses the TQM approach.

References

1. Deming, W. E., Quality, productivity and competitive positions (Cambridge, Mass.: MIT, 1982).
   WE Deming Out of Crisis (Cambridge Mass.: MIT, 1986).
2. Juran, J. M., *Quality Control Handbook*, 3rd edn (New York: Mc Graw-Hill, 1979).
3. NHS Management Executive, *The Quality Journey* (Lancs: Health Publications Ltd, 1993).

Further Reading

Berwick, D. M., 'Continuous improvement as an ideal in health care', *New England Medical Journal* (1989) **320**, 53.

Carr-Hill, R., *The NHS and Its Customers* (York Centre for Health Economics, University of York, 1989).

Feizenbaum, A. V., 'Total Quality Developments into the 1990s', in R. L. Chase (ed.) *TQM* (New York: IFS Publications, 19??).

Koch, H. C. H., *Training Manuals in TQM* (Brighton: Pavilion Publishing, 1991).

Koch, H. C. H., *Total Quality Management in Health Care* (Longman, 1991).

Oakland, J., *TQM* (Oxford: Heinemann, 1989).

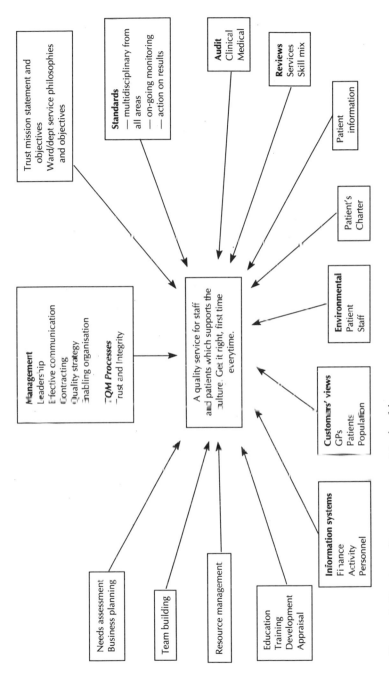

Trust mission statement and objectives
Ward/dept service philosophies and objectives

Standards
— multidisciplinary from all areas
— on-going monitoring
— action on results

Audit
Clinical
Medical

Reviews
Services
Skill mix

Patient information

Patient's Charter

Management
Leadership
Effective communication
Contracting
Quality strategy
Enabling organisation

TQM Processes
Trust and Integrity

A quality service for staff and patients which supports the culture. Get it right, first time everytime.

Environmental
Patient
Staff

Customers' views
GPs
Patients
Population

Information systems
Finance
Activity
Personnel

Needs assessment
Business planning

Team building

Resource management

Education
Training
Development
Appraisal

Figure 6 Total quality management in health care

Chapter 3 Standards of Care

Having written and agreed a philosophy and objectives as described in Chapter 1, the next step in the quality cycle is to describe the clinical care, or what we do, in measurable terms. Following this, to identify standards and criteria in order to establish the quality of patient care. It is not possible to measure the quality of care unless it has been accurately described in measurable terms. One of the ways to do this is by setting standards.

Background

There has been a great deal of standard-writing activity all over the United Kingdom. Some of the standards are excellent and there is evidence that the use of standards has improved patient care, but there are also areas where the activity is not so dynamic. On my visits around the country, in various guises, I ask to see the ward or department's standard of care. In some cases what can only be described as a tome of standards is lifted from the shelf, the dust blown off the cover and then handed to me. Within this large folder there may be dozens of standards, probably written by a manager or the lead person in quality assurance some time in the early 1980s. The staff can't tell you what the standards are about, when they are monitored or how they are used to monitor patient care. For standards to have an impact on patient care, they need to be written by the people who deliver care everyday, and to reflect current research-based practice.

There should only be about five or six current standards.

Once a standard is easily achieved it should be replaced by another standard that will improve patient care. The old standard may be reviewed occasionally and monitored to check that the outcomes are still being achieved.

Every member of staff should be involved in both the setting and the monitoring of the standards. Standards should reflect the expertise of the caring teams and the specific care required for the patient in that particular clinical area. Standards should be evidence based and dynamic – always moving, always changing to ensure or improve the quality of patient care – and not just a paper exercise. In order to make standards more dynamic I have further developed the system of standard-setting, and in particular the monitoring of standards, since the publication of the first edition of this book. In particular the monitoring of outcomes has become simpler, much more succint and part of everyday care, rather than formal monitoring on a planned basis – for example, every four or six months. This new approach is described in this next chapter.

The aim of this chapter is to enable you to set, write and monitor your own standards. The framework outlined is the one used by the Royal College of Nursing[1] which in turn is based on the Donabedian[2] triad. Although this framework has been used to set standards in nursing, it has also been used successfully by members of the professions allied to medicine, and other members of the health care team. It is very simple, straightforward and could be adapted to set standards anywhere.

By the time you have worked through this chapter you should have set a standard and developed a method by which to monitor it. The questions listed below are those that are most commonly asked during standards workshops and by the time you have completed this chapter you should have the answers to them.

- How do I choose a subject on which to write a standard?
- How many standards do I have to write?
- What good will it do – why bother?
- What is the difference between a standard, a policy and a procedure?
- How can I write standards or even think about standards

when we are short staffed, hard-pressed and under pressure?
- How can I monitor standards frequently?

This chapter has been designed to give you some background knowledge about quality assurance, where standards fit in to a quality assurance programme, and how to set, write and monitor standards. At the end of each section there is an exercise for you to complete so that by the time you have worked your way through the chapter you will have a standard, a method of monitoring and the knowledge and confidence to write some more standards for your own particular clinical area.

This chapter concentrates on setting and monitoring standards of care as a method of measuring the quality of patient care. In 1969, in the USA, Avedis Donabedian divided the evaluation of quality of care into the evaluation of the structure in which care is delivered, the process and the outcome of care (Donabedian, 1969).[2] Today his findings are still highly valued and form the basis of much of the work on quality assurance which is taking place all over the world.

What is quality assurance? Quality assurance is the measurement of the actual level of the service provided plus the efforts to modify, when necessary, the provision of these services in the light of the results of measurement.

Quality of care is the responsibility of everyone involved in health care and it was never more important than it is today. There are a variety of reasons for the ever-increasing focus on quality assurance. For example, the general public's expectations of the quality of care that they should receive has been raised through the publication of the Patient's Charter. Patients and relatives are encouraged to complain if the service is not satisfactory, and their views about the quality of care are actively sought by staff providing a service. There is also the presence of the 'press', ready to pick up on care and services that 'go wrong', with the resulting bad publicity for the organisation concerned.

The increasing competition within the internal market created by the NHS reforms has meant that managers and chief executives are facing major pressures for quality improvements which in turn are passed down through the organisation. Apart from these forces there is the professionals' desire to deliver good quality care for their patients.

Setting and monitoring standards of care and quality assurance are separate issues, although you may hear people discuss them as though they are the same. For example, it may be stated that standards are poor, implying that quality is poor and this leads to the misconception that standards and quality assurance are one and the same – but this is not the case. A standard is a *tool* to measure the quality of care as part of quality assurance.

What are Standards of Care?

Standards are valid, acceptable definitions of the quality of care. Standards cannot be valid unless they contain criteria to enable care to be measured and evaluated in terms of *effectiveness* and *quality*. Standards written without criteria can be likened to using a ruler without any measurements marked on it and then attempting a scale drawing: the 'measurements' would be an estimate and therefore inaccurate and variable.

Why do we Need Standards of Care?

Well written standards enable nurses, physiotherapists, chiropodists – in fact, anyone involved in health care – to describe in measurable terms the care they provide for patients, what is required to carry out that care and what the expected outcome will be. Perhaps in the past we have not been explicit about what we do and this has led to people from other backgrounds having a less than clear idea about our roles and responsibilities. In the late 1970s and early 1980s the health service, and in particular the nursing service, was faced with cut-backs and enormous change. The Royal College of Nursing was concerned about reduced numbers of nurses and falling standards, so a working group was set up to develop ways of measuring the quality of nursing care.

This group produced two documents: *Standards of Nursing Care* (1980)[3] and *Towards Standards* (1981).[4] Although these two documents apply specifically to nursing, they are equally applicable to the professions allied to medicine and other members of the health care team, as may be seen in the four main themes detailed below.

In *Standards of Nursing Care* four main themes were put forward:

1. Nurses should develop their own standards of care and the profession should agree on acceptable levels of excellence.
2. Good nursing is planned, systematic and focused on mutually agreed goals.
3. Agreed standards provide a base line for measurement.
4. Standards of care influence nursing practice, education, management and research.

In *Towards Standards* the working party identified eight prerequisites for successful, professional setting and control of standards of nursing care. (Again, these may be applied to other professions and members of the health care team.)

1. A philosophy of nursing
2. The relevant knowledge and skills
3. The nurse's authority to act
4. Accountability
5. The control of resources
6. The organisational structure and management style
7. The doctor–nurse relationship
8. The management of change.

In summary, the document identified the need for a statement of the underlying values and philosophy to guide nursing practice before quality nursing care could be assured. The philosophy had to be agreed and made explicit.

The following factors were linked with the philosophy:

- There must be clear identification of the skills and knowledge required by the nurse in order to carry out care effectively. The nurse must to be given the authority to act and be accountable for that action.
- Of the eight factors listed above, accountability is the key

to the formation of professional standards. Nurses must be clear about the extent of their authority, responsibility and accountability which must be matched with the necessary authority to carry out their job effectively.

The last four factors relate to the control of the nursing system.

Managers and senior nurses must be prepared to provide nurses with the appropriate manpower and equipment to do the job effectively. There must be a recognition of the nurses' need to control appropriate resources, to manage the service and to enjoy a relationship of mutual respect with other professionals. Finally, nurses must be in a position to initiate and manage change, a principle implicit in general management.

How can we use Standards?

Standards can be used to obtain information to:

- monitor care
- assess the level of service
- identify deficiencies
- communicate expectations
- introduce new knowledge
- make explicit what we do.

Exercise 3a

If possible get together with a group of your colleagues and go through the questions at the beginning of this chapter. See if you have the answers to any of the questions and make a note of those left unanswered. Then check these off as you work your way through the rest of this chapter.

The Quality Assurance Cycle

It is important to understand where standards fit into the quality assurance cycle (see Figure 7). It has always been very difficult to describe care in measurable terms but standards help us to do just that.

1. Describing

The first part of the cycle is the 'describing' part and it is helpful to start by writing a philosophy of care, as described in Chapter 1. This is really a statement about what we believe we are doing to help and care for our patients or clients – Why are we here? What do we believe we are doing? This does not have to be a highly academic statement but should be a few words that describe what you believe you are doing. From this will come your objectives – what you hope to achieve. Once you have written your philosophy and objectives then it will become apparent what standards you will need to write

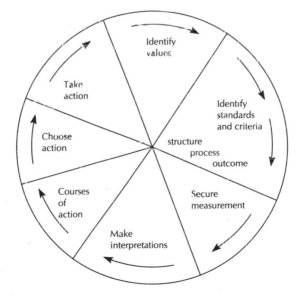

Figure 7 The quality assurance cycle

in order to measure the effectiveness of your philosophy and objectives. So the first step is to describe what you do in measurable terms, and then to identify standards and criteria in order to establish the quality of service.

2. Measuring

The next part of the cycle is measuring the standards. It is not possible to measure the quality of care unless it has been accurately described in measurable terms.

Once the standard has been measured, the results should be reviewed, criteria not achieved should be identified and interpretations made about compliance with the standard.

3. Taking action

The last and most important step is taking action – comparing what should be with what is and taking action to ensure that the quality of care is assured.

Then go round the cycle again to ensure improvements were made.

Who Writes the Standards?

Standards are written by staff working in clinical areas. They are written on topics that they select, and are relevant to the needs of both staff and clients. Standards are often written to solve a problem but they may also be written for an area of concern or one of particular interest or good practice.

Being involved in setting and monitoring standards of care means being committed to looking at what you do and being prepared to take the appropriate action to change things to improve the quality of patient care. All standards should be research-based, which means establishing sound reasons for practice and taking an extra look at what you do – not giving care that is ritualistic, unnecessary or of no proven value.

Exercise 3b

If you are working in a group, then discuss the following questions. If you are on your own, list your answers to them.

1. Why is it important to be able to describe what you do?
2. How do you measure the quality of care that you give to your patients or clients?
3. How do you get yourself to take an extra look at what you do?

Levels of Standard Setting and Monitoring

There are various levels of standard setting, as shown in Figure 8.

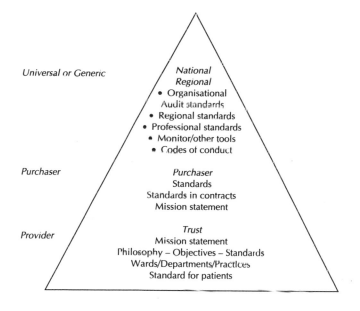

Figure 8 Levels of standard setting and monitoring

1. Universal or generic

This level is related to the profession's philosophy of care, what the profession believes about caring for patients or clients. Standards at this level relate to mission statements and a professional code of conduct. The UKCC professional code of conduct for nurses identifies fourteen different categories which are useful as guidelines for clinical practice. Although they could not be used in a ward or clinical area to measure the quality of care, they must be in the system to ensure good practice.

This level also includes standards written at Regional level by the Regional Health Authority for a particular service such as nursing, physiotherapy, occupational therapy, chiropody.

Also at this level are the various national audits, such as Organisational Audit and the Audit Commission. (See Chapter 1 for more details.)

2. Purchaser level

At this level there may be specific purchasing standards which the purchaser expects all providers to achieve. On the other hand, the contract should contain indicators of quality which are part of the contractual agreement and must be conformed with. The quality issues with the contract may focus on the Health of the Nation targets, the 'Patient's Charter' or areas of concern identified by the consumer. The purchaser will also focus on issues and trends which have arisen from national studies.

This level is important as it demonstrates the direction the provider is expected to develop and move. These levels of standard setting and measurement of quality will not necessarily translate themselves directly into the way that care is delivered on the wards and in departments, but they are essential and they need to be adapted to reflect local performance.

3. Provider level

Local standards are developed by professionals or any member of the health care team working in a particular area or with a specific care group. These standards are statements that are specific and about activities in wards and units.

They are presented in statements of performance to be achieved within an agreed time and are: *acceptable, achievable, observable* and *measurable*. This is the level at which standards are set in wards, departments, geographical areas of Community Trusts and locally based units.

Exercise 3c

If you are working in a group, then discuss the following questions. If you are working on your own, then list the answers.

1. Has anyone set standards in your hospital or in the area in which you work?
2. Where are these standards kept?
3. Has your Regional Health Authority set any standards?
4. Has your professional organisation set any standards?
5. Has there been an organisational audit? If so, who undertook the audit and what were the results?

Terminology Used in Standard Setting

There is an enormous amount of 'jargon' used in the setting and monitoring of standards, but in order to write standards it is important to understand the terminology.

1. A standard statement

Standard statements are professionally agreed levels of performance, appropriate to the population addressed, which reflect what is *acceptable, observable, achievable* and *measurable*. The first part of the statement, 'Standard statements are professionally agreed', means that a group of professionals or members of the health care team get together and in discussion agree a standard, taking into account research findings and changes in practice.

The first and vital step in standard setting is the beginning of the provision of continuity of care for the patient. The discussions about 'what we do' and 'who does it' prior to setting the standard are very valuable. These discussions may identify duplication of effort by professionals, differences in the way care is given and a debate on what should be done by whom, how and when.

The standard statement should include the indicators of quality. For example: 'Every resident chooses and wears their own clothes at all times' – Why? So what? The indicator of quality is 'In order to promote dignity and self respect'.

Residents who are dressed by staff in clothes from a general stock of clothes are given no choice. This is a very poor indicator of quality: their dignity has been removed, they have become institutionalised. The standard is written and implemented to ensure that all residents are enabled to retain their self respect, dignity and right to choice.

The second part of the statement, 'Related to a level of performance', means establishing what you are trying to achieve for your patients/clients within your resources, and reaching the desired outcome. 'Appropriate to the population addressed', means the care group for which the standard is written, taking into account the patient's/client's and relative's needs, negotiating care with patients/clients, developing shared plans of care. The standard may be written for children or patients admitted for surgery, and so on.

2. Criteria

Criteria may be defined as descriptive statements of performance, behaviours, circumstances or clinical status that represent a satisfactory, positive or excellent state of affairs.

A criterion is a variable, or item, that is selected as a relevant indicator of the quality of care.

Criteria make the standard work because they are detailed indicators of the standard and must be specified to the area or type of patient.

Criteria must be:

- **measurable** – illustrating the standard and providing local measures
- **specific** – giving a clear description of behaviours/action/situation/resources desired or required
- **relevant** – items that you can identify that are required in

order to achieve a set level of performance. There may be numerous criteria that you can think of, but you have to learn to be selective and pick out only those criteria that are the relevant indicators of quality of care and which must be met in order to achieve a set level of performance

- **clearly understandable** – therefore they should each contain only one major theme or thought
- **clearly and simply stated** so as to avoid being misunderstood
- **achievable** – it is important to avoid unrealistic expectations in either performance or results
- **clinically sound** – therefore they must be selected by practitioners who are clinically up to date and evidence based
- **reviewed periodically** – to ensure that they are reflective of good practice based on current research
- **reflective of all aspects of the patient or client status** – that is physiological, psychological and social.

In summary, a criterion must be:

- a detailed indicator of the standard
- specific to the area and type of patient or client
- measurable.

Think of the standard as a tape measure or ruler and the criteria as the measurement marks. The criteria allow you to measure the standard, they make it possible to measure the standard statement.

There are three types of criteria:

- *structure*
- *process*
- *outcome.*

2.1 Structure criteria

Structure criteria describe what must be provided in order to achieve the standard – the items of service which are in the system, such as:

- the physical environment and buildings
- ancillary and support services
- equipment

- staff: numbers, skill, mix, training, expertise
- information: agreed policies and procedures, rules and regulations
- organisational system.

2.2 Process criteria

Process criteria describe what action must take place in order to achieve the standard:

- the assessment techniques and procedures
- methods of delivery of care
- the assessment procedure
- methods of intervention
- methods of patient, client, relative and/or carer education
- methods of giving information
- methods of documenting
- how resources are used
- evaluation of the competence of staff carrying out the care.

The following headings indicate the areas to include in process criteria.

The professional assesses . . .
The professional includes in the plan . . .
The professional does . . .
The professional reviews . . .
The professional and the patient or client . . .

2.3 Outcome criteria

Outcome criteria describe the effect of the care – the results expected in order to achieve the standard in terms of behaviours, responses, level of knowledge and health status. In other words, what is expected and desirable described in a specific and measurable form.

Consider the following headings:

The nurse can state . . .
The patient can state . . .
There is documented evidence . . .
The professional observed . . .

One of the reasons for developing the outcome criteria into immediately measurable criteria is to ensure that standards are measured all the time as part of the evaluation of care. Many professionals see the measurement of standards as 'someone else's responsibility', rather than part of patient or client care. Outcomes that are not being achieved need to be corrected immediately, not left for quarterly or six-monthly formal monitoring.

In summary, criteria state:

- what we need to meet the standard
- what must be done to meet the standard
- expected results or outcome. (See Figure 9.)

Structure	Process	Outcome
Resource	Action	Results
What you need	What has to be done	Outcome

Figure 9 Criteria: a summary

In the past the outcomes set were very broad criteria, for example: 'the discharge was carried out in accordance with the individual's needs and wishes'. This outcome requires a monitoring tool in order to measure the patient's satisfaction. It is much simpler to state:

Outcome   YES NO

- The patient can state:
  — that the discharge plan was discussed   ☑   ☐
  with him/her
  — the discharge plan.   ☑   ☐

- There was a documented assessment of   ☑   ☐
  the patient's needs prior to discharge

It is important to remember that the criteria describe the *activities* to be performed, whereas the standard states the *level* at which they are to be performed. The criteria are like the strings on a puppet, making the standards come alive. By following this process, patient or client care can be measured by comparing actual practice against the stated criteria and then checking to see if the activity has met the agreed standard.

Classifying Standards

This method of writing standards is a dynamic approach, as it involves writing standards about an area of interest or concern, or in order to solve a problem. As you can imagine, this could lead to vast amounts of information and there is a danger of overwhelming the system. In order to organise the information, Helen Kendall of West Berkshire Health Authority[5] devised a simple format to co-ordinate the information. Every standard must be classified according to the following headings.

1. Topic

This is a major activity classified according to a particular coding system (see Figure 10). The area of interest, concern, or the problem on which you have decided to write your standard, can be located under one of these topics. For example, a standard being written to solve a problem transferring patients from a hospital to the community would be 'continuity of care'.

2. Sub-Topic

This is a sub-system of classifications which enables you to define further the area of interest, concern or problem. So, if the topic is 'continuity of care', and the sub-topic is 'transfer of patient', the problem concerns the transfer of patients or clients (see Figure 10).

The form in Figure 11 is used to record all standards and is based on one designed by Helen Kendall. This is an example of the type of form used and you may need to use some or all

Standards of Care

TOPIC	SUB-TOPIC
Patient/Client	
SAFETY	ELIMINATING HAZARDS THEATRE STANDARDS CONTROL OF INFECTION STANDARD
INDIVIDUALISED CARE	SYSTEMATIC APPROACH
ACTIVITIES OF DAILY LIVING	MAINTAINING A SAFE ENVIRONMENT COMMUNICATING
(i) 'PHYSICAL'	BREATHING EATING AND DRINKING ELIMINATING
(ii) 'PSYCHOLOGICAL'	PERSONAL CLEANSING AND DRESSING CONTROLLING BODY TEMPERATURE MOBILISING WORKING AND PLAYING EXPRESSING SEXUALITY SLEEPING DYING PAIN
CONTINUITY OF CARE	RECEPTION/ADMISSION OF PATIENTS OR CLIENTS DISCHARGE OF PATIENTS TRANSFER OF PATIENTS
INDEPENDENCE AND INVOLVEMENT	PROMOTION OF SELF-CARE DECISIONS/CHOICES ABILITY TO CARE FOR SELF REHABILITATION FAMILY/CARER PARTICIPATION
PRIVACY AND CONFIDENTIALITY	PRIVACY – ENVIRONMENT AND ATTITUDES TO PRIVACY ACCESS TO RECORDS
Staff/Other	
PERSONNEL	SELECTION/INTERVIEWING RECRUITMENT
BASIC AND CONTINUING EDUCATION AND APPRAISAL	COMPETENCES ORIENTATION PROGRAMMES PROFESSIONAL DEVELOPMENT

Source: Based on a form designed by Helen Kendall.

Figure 10 Topics and sub-topics

of the headings. Topic and sub-topic have already been discussed above. The explanation of the rest of the form is as follows.

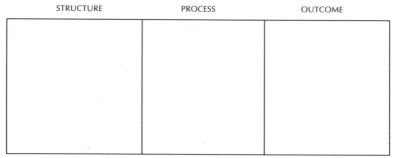

STANDARD REF NO. ....   ACHIEVED STANDARD BY ....

TOPIC ....   REVIEW STANDARD BY ....

SUB-TOPIC ....   SIGNATURE OF FACILITATOR ....

CARE GROUP ....   SIGNATURE OF MANAGER ....

CLINICAL AREA ....   DATE STANDARD SET ....

MONITORING RESULTS ....   DATE TO BE MONITORED ....

           DATE OF MONITORING ....

STANDARD STATEMENT ....

....

STRUCTURE	PROCESS	OUTCOME

Figure 11   Form for recording standards

3. Standard reference number

In the top left-hand corner there is the 'Standard Reference Number' – this is where the index number is recorded. An index system is used to organise the information and make it quick and simple to find standards and share them with any-one who would like to see them. It is easy to pull them up by topic, sub-topic, care group, clinical area, review-by date and monitoring result. If anyone is having problems writing a stan-dard, they can ask for a copy of those that have already been written and this helps them to get started.

4. Care group

This is the target group of patients, clients or staff for whom the standard is written, such as 'care of the elderly', 'patients in the recovery room', patients with a specific problem, such as diabetes or those recovering from a cerebral vascular accident, 'mother and baby', 'children', 'patients or clients in the community', and so on.

5. Clinical area

This is the ward, unit, department locally-based unit, clinic, surgery and soon.

6. Achieve by date and review by date

It is important to decide when the standard will be achieved and to set and record a realistic date. You will also need to discuss and decide when it would be reasonable to review the standard and decide if it is still relevant, achievable, acceptable, and in line with current practice and research. If it is not, then it should be removed from the system and replaced by an appropriate standard. It is important to realise that standards set today are not set in tablets of stone forever but are reviewed and rewritten; they are dynamic and change as the patient's or client's needs change, as new research changes practice, as patients or clients change, or as staff change.

7. Facilitator's signature

The person who has been trained to facilitate the process of setting standards signs here. In West Dorset we trained fifty people, who were selected to represent the clinical areas throughout the district. These people were given training to enable them to work with groups, set and monitor standards and facilitate their colleagues in the clinical areas.

8. Manager's signature

The manager signs the standard statement to say that he or she agrees that the content is acceptable, observable, measurable, applicable to the group specified and achievable in the particular unit by the specified date.

9. Result of monitoring

Here 'achieved' or 'not achieved' is written. If the standard has not been achieved, then an action plan should be developed to ensure achievement.

Classifying standards in this way helps to keep them succinct and clearly focused on a particular care group.

The good news is that standards should only be a page long. If they go on for longer, then you may well be rewriting the procedure book. It is very easy to write down everything that you can think of in relation to a problem, but more difficult to be succinct and only include the indicators of quality.

Checking Standards

Once you have written the standard, check that the criteria:

- describe the desired quality of performance
- have been agreed
- are clearly written (not open to misinterpretation)
- contain only one major thought
- are measurable
- are concise
- are specific
- are achievable
- are clinically sound.

Monitoring Standards

There are two approaches to monitoring standards, through:

- retrospective evaluation
- concurrent evaluation

Retrospective evaluation involves all assessment methods that occur after the patient or client has been discharged. Concurrent evaluation involves assessment that takes place while the patient or client is still receiving care. Figure 12 lists the

Exercise 3d

Get together in a group, in your clinical area, and set a standard using the framework described in this chapter. This group may consist of people from one profession, such as nursing, or it may be the multidisciplinary team caring for a group of patients or clients. Consider these points:

1. Is there someone with experience of setting standards available to help you with this activity?
2. Ensure your manager knows what you are doing and see if he or she would like to be involved.
3. Set a time limit on the group's activity and decide when to meet again and what you hope to achieve.
4. Select a topic. When selecting a topic, bear in mind the following points.

- Can you agree on the area of interest, concern or problem on which you would like to set a standard?
- Can you realistically solve the problem that you have selected?
- How much work and time will you have to commit to this exercise?
- Will the end result improve patient care?
- Write down all the ideas associated with the problem or area of concern or interest and identify those that fall into structure, process and outcome criteria.
- Can you agree a standard?
- Having agreed a standard statement, is it easier to work across the criteria so that there is a link between structure, process and outcome? Or is it simpler to list all the structure, then all the process, and then the outcome criteria?
- Is it easier to write the outcome criteria first and work backwards?
- Are the criteria measurable?
- Are the criteria the indicators of quality?
- Do the structure, process and outcome criteria measure the standard statement?
- How will you monitor the standard?
- When should it be achieved? Remember, be realistic about this date.
- When should the standard be reviewed – after three months, six months, a year?
- Discuss the completed standard with your manager.

Retrospective evaluation of the quality of nursing care may be effected by:	Concurrent evaluation may be effected by:

Post-care patient interview
Post-care patient questionnaire
Post-care staff conference
Audit of the records
	Assessment of the outcome
	Patient interview
	Conference between patient,
	   staff and relatives
	Direct observation of care
	Measurement of the
	  competency of the nurse
	Audit of the records

Figure 12 Retrospective and concurrent evaluation of care

YES	NO	N/A	MONITORING STANDARDS

			Retrospective/Concurrent evaluation
			Questions to be answered
			Developed from the criteria in the standard
			Auditor checks the criteria in question
			form:
			
			● Asks the patient about care received
			● Asks the staff about care given
			● Observes care given/structure of area
			  and reviews documentation
			● Responds by answering Yes/No/Not
			  applicable
			
			RESPONSE SHOULD BE 100% 'YES'. ANY
			'NO' ANSWERS SHOULD BE
			INVESTIGATED AND AN ACTION PLAN
			DEVELOPED; A DATE SHOULD BE SET TO
			RE-MONITOR STANDARDS.

Figure 13 Monitoring standards using retrospective and concurrent evaluation

approaches used to assess the quality of care. The use of concurrent evaluation is perhaps more valuable, as it gives staff the opportunity to correct any negative outcomes while the patient is still in their care. This approach is further developed in Figure 13.

When monitoring standards or when establishing patient, client or relative views it is sometimes necessary to develop questionnaires, as discussed later on in this chapter, on p. 60.

1. Approaches to monitoring standards

1.1 Type 1

As discussed earlier, the process of monitoring standards may be made simpler and more effective by writing the outcome criteria in a form that requires a 'yes' or 'no' answer. Remember that each outcome criterion must contain only one question or theme.

Example 1

OUTCOME
The patient can state that his discharge plan was negotiated with him and met his identified needs.

In responding to this outcome you could say 'yes' the plan met his needs but it was *not* negotiated with him.
   To turn this into an outcome that is measurable, you could put it in this form:

The patient can state   YES   NO

- his or her discharge plan   ☑   ☐
- his or her discharge plan was negotiated with him/her   ☑   ☐
- the plan meets his or her assessed needs.   ☑   ☐

This standard can be measured every time a patient is discharged by simply including the outcomes in the discharge plan check list or in the care plan. Any negatives would be reported, noted and action taken to correct them.
   If the outcome criteria have not been met then the next step would be to establish why it was not met, by going back through the process and the structure to establish what went wrong, then putting it right by taking action immediately.

1.2 Type 2

An alternative approach is to take criteria from structure, process and outcome and turn them into a list of questions. Each question is used as an indicator which requires a 'yes' or 'no' answer. The total number of 'yes' answers may be added together to calculate a score and demonstrate whether or not the standard has been achieved.

2. Methods of monitoring standards

There are various methods of monitoring standards, of which the most commonly used are:

- observation of care
- asking the patient, client or relative questions
- checking the records.

The various types of measurement need to be discussed by the group and the most appropriate method selected.

2.1 Questionnaires

The techniques for asking questions have been thoroughly researched and there are many different approaches. Payne[6], Maccoby *et al.*,[7] Gorden[8] and Oppenheim[9] all have excellent discussions on the art of asking questions. Ward *et al.*[10] give many examples of different approaches to patient surveys. From these findings and recommendations, the following points arise.

- Questions should be phrased so they do not patronise the respondent, while at the same time being easily understood, and so meet the intellectual abilities of a cross section of society.
- Questions must be expressed simply and clearly, making sure not to use words and phrases that have more than one meaning.
- Ask questions one at a time. Do not include two topics in one question – for example: 'was your discharge planned and negotiated with you?' The care may have been planned with the patient but not necessarily negotiated. Ask two separate questions, as the answers could be very different.

- Questions should be short.
- Give the respondent an opportunity to write his or her comments.
- Respondents tend to choose a middle answer if given a choice so a simple 'yes' or 'no' will overcome this problem.
- Sometimes a respondent may show a bias by answering 'yes' to every question. To avoid this you can ask a question where a positive answer is required and then later in the questionnaire ask the same or a similar question where a negative response is required. Including different forms of the same question can also check for consistency and misunderstandings.

These are only a few suggestions, but they may help you when you come to prepare a questionnaire to monitor a standard.

2.2 The care plan

The patient's or client's care plan is a very effective method of monitoring when a standard that is written for a group of patients or clients is monitored for an individual.

The Final Stage

The final stage in standard setting is to compare current practice with the standard and to act on the monitoring result. If the standard has not been achieved, you need to check why. Ask yourself: Is it an achievable standard? Is it realistic? If not, review the standard. If it is achievable, then develop an action plan to ensure that practice meets the standard.

As demonstrated in Figure 14, the measurement of standards is not 'quality assured'. Quality assurance only occurs when the gaps have been identified following measurement, and action has been taken to ensure standards are achieved.

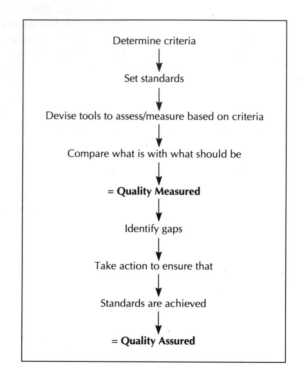

Figure 14 Quality measured. Quality assured

Summary of Points on Standard Setting

- When writing a standard, start with the standard statement.
- Then identify the outcome criteria in question form, ready to monitor.
- Then identify the process required to achieve the outcome (what must be done)
- Then identify the structure – what we need to deliver the process to meet the pre-set outcome
- Be succinct: you are a group of professionals who work together all the time and the process criteria should not develop into the procedure book. Identify key criteria.
- Use only words that are measurable – for example, you cannot measure 'as required,' 'as necessary', 'understands', 'appropriate'. You need to identify what words mean in measurable terms. For example, if you say: 'The patient understands his medication', how do you know this? A simple, measurable way of stating this might be:

The patient can state:

	YES	NO
• the time medication is to be taken	☑	☐
• the dosage of medication	☑	☐
• the side-effects of medication	☑	☐

- Check that the outcomes measure the standard statement.
- Involve the multidisciplinary team in setting standards.
- Monitoring standards should be a part of patient care evaluation.
- Standards should reflect the specialised care required by your patients.
- Standards should be taken out of the system once they have been easily achieved – put on the shelf, and reviewed in a few months to check they are still being achieved. New standards should be brought in to improve patient care.

It is important to remember that standards written at local level are written by those who are giving the care. The very process of setting standards leads to discussion about practice: who does what and how. In any team of professionals there will be a variety of people, all of whom were trained at different times, and have varying amounts of experience and competence.

Talking about practice gives everyone a chance to share experience and expertise and this alone improves the quality of care. In order to have an agreed standard there must be consensus of opinion which inevitably leads to continuity of care.

Continuity of care, practising according to research findings and keeping up to date can be a potential problem, particularly for professionals working in isolation, and the process of setting standards is a very useful method of promoting good quality care.

When I have discussed standard setting with groups of professionals, one problem that is always mentioned is the lack of time that they have available to set standards, particularly as a multidisciplinary team. One solution to the problem that seems to go down well is the 'little and often principle', as follows.

Try to use time when you already routinely meet. Most wards or departments meet to discuss patient care, either for a report on patient care or at a case conference. At the end of these meetings, spend literally a few minutes setting standards. Here is an example of how this might be done.

- At the first meeting, discuss what the topic of the standard might be. Write your thoughts on a large piece of paper and leave it for anyone who was not there that day to add their thoughts.
- At the next meeting, try to draft the standard statement; again, write it up and leave it for comments.
- At the next meeting, try to establish the outcome criteria.
- Then at following meetings add the process and the structure.

Using this approach means that all members of staff are involved. Everyone in the team contributes to the standard. During the short sessions there are opportunities to discuss the content of the standard. Everyone agrees the standard and has a clear understanding of the monitoring approach. As a result, at the end of the process there will be a commitment to the standard and possibly changes in practice that will have already improved patient care.

It is advisable to set a few standards, perhaps five or six, so it is not an enormous task. Of course the standards will need to be changed when they are easily achieved, to ensure a continuous improvement of patient care. For example, if a ward or department sets five key standards, and one is easily achieved, then it should be put on the shelf and a new standard established on another topic, perhaps in response to an area where care could be improved. The standard on the shelf should be monitored occasionally to ensure it is still being achieved, and it should be brought back into the system if this is not the case.

The following example of standards have been written for a variety of reasons.

Example 2 demonstrates how outcome criteria are used as the monitoring tool as part of the evaluation of patient care – ongoing monitoring.

Example 2

A problem where there is poor follow-up of patients referred to the community nurses.

Standard statement: Each patient is visited by a community nurse within 24 hours of referral.

In order to meet this standard, there are some essential structure, process and outcome criteria:

Structure criteria:
● Contact point at GP surgery or health centre for receiving messages:
● Nursing history forms available.

Process criteria:
● The nurse visits the contact point every morning and registers messages received;
● The nurse visits and assesses the patient's needs within 24 hours;
● The nurse ensures that the patient understands and agrees the plan of care;
● The nurse records the visit in the patient's home notes.

Outcome criteria:
● The nurse visited within 24 hours of referral (documented evidence)
● The patient states that his or her individual needs are being met (ask patient)
● Forms are completed (documented evidence)
● Assessment is completed (documented evidence)
● Assessment is completed within 24 hours (documented evidence)

Example 3 is a standard written in response to a problem concerning staff safety. Staff have received an injury from disposed, used sharps.

Example 3

Standard statement: All sharps will be disposed of without injury to members of staff.

In order to meet this standard, there are some essential structure, process and outcome criteria:

Structure criteria:
- District policy on disposal of sharps;
- Education for staff;
- Staff have knowledge of this policy.
- Sharps safe box; polythene bag and label.

Process criteria:
- The professional places all used sharps in the sharps safe box immediately.
- The container is closed when it is three-quarters full.
- The container is placed in a polythene bag and labelled 'for incineration'.

Outcome criteria:
- All sharps are successfully incinerated (ask staff responsible).
- There are no injuries to staff from sharps (documentary evidence).

The 'snap shot' monitoring of this standard might lead to results that indicate a serious problem which necessitates the setting up of an audit to resolve the problem. Clinical audit is described in Chapter 4. Example 4 demonstrates how a standard may be monitored for all patients as part of their care.

Example 4:

Topic: Continuity of care

Subtopic: Discharge from hospital

Care group: Patients nursed on a medical ward

Standard statement: Each patient's discharge is planned in accordance with his or her wishes and needs by the multidisciplinary team to ensure continuity of care.

Structure criteria:
- Patient's individual assessment forms and care plans;

- Professional has knowledge of services in the community.
- Checklist for services;
- Patient information booklets;
- Multidisciplinary team.

Process criteria:
- The professional (key worker) carries out an ongoing assessment of the patient's needs.
- The professional (key worker) co-ordinates the discharge information and relays it to other agencies and services.
- The professional (key worker) completes the checklist;
- The professional (key worker) educates the patient, using information leaflets and instructions.

Outcome criteria:
- There is a completed discharge plan.
- The discharge plan is acceptable to the patient and relatives.
- All support services have been arranged.
- Discharge check list is completed.
- The patient is able to describe his or her medical/nursing/therapy needs at home.

Monitoring of this standard may be carried out by:
- Checking that the patient's assessment is complete and that the care plan outlines the discharge plan;
- Checking that the checklist is completed;
- Asking the patient some key questions about his or her care and through discussion checking his or her understanding of the plan. For example:
  - Was your discharge plan started at least 48 hours before your discharge   YES/NO
  - Was your discharge planned with you   YES/NO
  - Was your discharge plan negotiated with you?   YES/NO
  - Does the plan meet your needs?   YES/NO
  - Did you receive written instruction about your care?   YES/NO
  - Has the checklist has been completed?   YES/NO

On the other hand, the outcome could have been written as follows:

Outcome	YES	NO
The patient can state:		
● the plan for discharge	☑	☐
● the plan was acceptable	☑	☐
● his or her care at home	☑	☐
There is documented evidence:		
● of a documented discharge plan	☑	☐
● of a completed discharge checklist	☑	☐
● that all support services were arranged	☑	☐

Monitoring standards may be seen as taking a 'snap shot' of the quality of care to establish the standard of care. If the standard is poor, or there are problems, then there may be a need to develop an audit around the problem area, to thoroughly investigate the problem and identify and implement the solutions.

So you might see the monitoring of standards as a 'snap shot' of activity and the process of audit as a 'detailed portrait'.

Exercise 3e

Develop a method of monitoring the standard that you have already written.

References

1. Kitson, A., 'Indicators of quality in nursing care – an alternative approach', *Journal of Advanced Nursing* (1986) **11**, 133–44.
2. Donabedian, A., 'Evaluating the Quality of Medical Care', *Hilbank Memorial Fund Quarterly* (1969) **44**(2), 166–206.
3. Royal College of Nursing, *Standards of Nursing Care* (London, 1980).
4. Royal College of Nursing, *Towards Standards* (London, 1981).
5. Kendall, H., 'The West Berkshire Approach', *Nursing Times* (1988) **84**(27), 33–4.
6. Payne, S. I., *The Art of Asking Questions* (Princeton University Press, 1951).
7. Maccoby, E., *et al.*, 'The Interview: A Tool of Social Science', in *Handbook of Social Psychology*, vol. 1, *Theory and Method*, ed. G. Lindzey (Reading, Mass.: Addison-Wesley Publishing Company Inc., 1968).
8. Gorden, R. I., *Interviewing Strategy: Techniques and Tactics* (Homewood, Ill.: The Dorsey Press, 1969).
9. Oppenheim, A. N., *Questionnaire Design and Attitude Measurement* (London: Heinemann, 1979).
10. Ward, M. J., *et al.*, *Instruments for Measuring Practice and Other Health Care Variables*, vols 1 and 2 (Boulder, Colo.: Western Interstate Commission for Higher Education, 1982).

Further Reading

Cuthbert, M., 'Evaluating Patient Care', *Australian Nurses Journal* (1984) **13**(8).

Donabedian, A., *The Definition of Quality and Approaches to its Assessment*, vol. 1 (Health Administration Press, 1980).

Howell, J. and H. Marr, 'Raising the standards', *Nursing Times* (1988) **84**(25).

Kendall, H. and A. Kitson, 'Rest Assured', *Nursing Times* (1986) **82**(35), 28–31.

Kitson, A., 'Raising the standards', *Nursing Times* (1988) **84**(25), 28–32.

Lang, N., 'Issues in Quality Assurance in Nursing', *ANA Issues in Evaluation Research* (1976).

Sale, D. N. T., 'Participating in Standard Setting: Planning a Programme of Change', *International Journal of Health Care Quality Assurance* (1989) **2**(2).

Sale, D. N. T., 'Raising the standards – Down Dorset Way', *Nursing Times* (1988) **84**(28), 31 2.

Chapter 4   Clinical Audit

Definition

Clinical audit is a simple system which allows professionals to measure their performance, to recognise good practice and if necessary make improvements. The definition of audit presented in the 1989 White Paper was 'The systematic critical analysis of the quality of medical care, including the procedures used for diagnosis and treatment, the use of resources and the resulting outcome and quality of life for the patient.'

A clinical audit is not undertaken in isolation by one professional but is developed with the help of colleagues and the support of management. Clinical audit is an essential part of the desire to deliver quality of care by every professional involved in patient care.

The Audit Cycle

The audit process is a cycle not dissimilar from the quality assurance cycle as shown in Figure 15.

1. Observe current practice

As indicated in Figure 15, the first part of the cycle is to observe current practice and make an assessment of the quality of current practice.

71

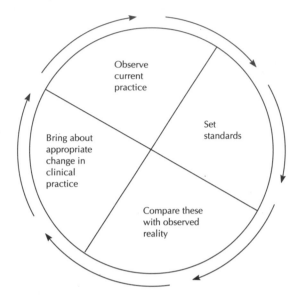

Figure 15 The audit process is a cycle

2. Set standards of care

The setting of standards is often seen as a difficult part of the cycle and is discussed in detail in Chapter 3.

3. Compare expectations with reality

The next part of the cycle is to compare expectations with observed reality. Having established what the standards are, there is a need to compare these with clinical practice. What is the reality? Where are the gaps? Is there a difference between standards which were set and the standards that actually take place when patient care is delivered? Having monitored the standards and identified the gap, then make comparisons. This will form the body of the clinical audit which will be described in more detail further on in this chapter.

4. Bring about appropriate change

This part of the cycle is perhaps the most important, because this is about making appropriate change, if it is required. If changes have been identified, then these need to be agreed with your colleagues. Changes in practice need to be carefully reviewed to ensure that they will result in the improvement of patient care. Having set up and implemented the changes, then monitor the changes. Observe the effects and improvements and whether there are any problems associated with making those changes.

Why do we need Clinical Audit?

Clinical audit gives professionals the opportunity to review clinical practice, to take a step back, to look at how care is delivered and the effects that care has on the patient and whether or not this can be improved. It also gives professionals an opportunity to monitor the effects that care has on patients. As professionals, I believe that we have always undertaken activities like this but perhaps not using a structured approach and certainly not as a multidisciplinary team. Having used the clinical audit process to monitor the effect of care given to patients, there is an opportunity to take note of the results and to change delivery of care. This is a chance to look at how things might be improved, how high quality care might be delivered, in a different way, in a more effective way that will benefit the patient.

Benefits

As stated above, this is an opportunity to question practice. Do staff continue to do things the way they have always been done? The answer to that is possibly 'yes' because there isn't time to review it and do it differently, but this is an opportunity to develop practice to move forward.

Benefits

- From the patient's point of view, this will lead to greater continuity of care from the multidisciplinary team.
- By looking at better ways of delivering care, we have an opportunity to raise the overall quality of care to a consistently higher level and constantly to improve the delivery of patient care.
- Clinical audit gives us an opportunity to reduce the number of clinical errors by looking at practice and identifying ways of delivering care that prevent mistakes and errors occurring.
- Through clinical audit it is possible to review the skills that staff have and how they are used, as they are often misplaced or misused.
- Clinical audit allows us to review the delivery of ineffective treatment where previously there has not been the opportunity to review what is and is not effective.
- As a result of clinical audit, changes in practice may save time. This time may then be used more appropriately in areas that require specialised professionals skills.
- The resulting changes to practice and delivery of care may well improve cost efficiency. Often the cost of poor quality care is significantly higher than the cost of delivering high quality care 'right first time'.
- Clinical audit gives professionals the opportunity to develop their own standards. This is important because it gives the staff a sense of 'owning' their owns standards of care that reflect efficient, effective good quality care being delivered to patients.
- Clinical audit also encourages self-improvement, taking that longer look at what we do, how we do it and asking could it be done better.
- If clinical audit is undertaken as a multidisciplinary team, this approach can lead to a greater understanding of how professionals perform in their own specialities and where the overlaps are in the delivery of care between the different members of the team. It gives staff an opportunity to identify who is best suited to deliver certain aspects of care and to work as an effective team, rather than as separate individuals.

Four Main Principles

Essentially there are four main principles to the development of the clinical audit, and these are applicable to any clinical area and any professional group, be it single discipline or multidisciplinary.

1. Define the objectives

It is important to remember that any effective care requires individuals to work as a team and depends on that team holding the same values and expectations to avoid the confusion created by people working to different objectives.

So the first step under this particular principle is to identify the mission statement of the organisation, and write the philosophy of care for the particular area in which your team is working. (See Chapter 3 for advice on writing a philosophy of care.)

Having undertaken this exercise and identified the philosophy of care for a particular area, the next step is to identify the key objectives of the service. Many areas will already have been through this process while undertaking a 'Setting of Standards' exercise a few years ago, so this will just be a continuation of the work that has already been undertaken. It is important to:

- keep the philosophy simple
- keep it general
- keep in mind the people for whom the philosophy is written — essentially, the patient and the patient's relatives.

It is always good to see philosophies (whether written by the multidisciplinary team or by individual groups of professionals) printed, published and hung up in the ward or department where patients and relatives may share the philosophy and be part of the approach to caring for them.

2. Develop standards and ways to measure them

Many professionals have already written their standards, and audit may be seen as a link between standard setting and more in-depth monitoring of quality and audit. As discussed in Chapter 3, it is important to understand the 'jargon' and the words that are used, so that areas of quality are not muddled. If professionals talk about auditing standards instead of monitoring standards, it gives the impression that every standard needs to be audited in depth, which of course is not true.

The monitoring of standards should be seen as a 'snapshot'

of activity, looking at whether or not standards are complied with and good quality care is achieved. If there is an area within those standards that the staff are having difficulty achieving, then this may be the area that is pulled out and developed for clinical audit. In other words, audit should be seen to be a 'detailed portrait' of the area of activity being monitored, and monitoring of standards should be seen as a simple 'snapshot'. If, on the other hand, the organisation does not have standards at this point and you are embarking on clinical audit, then this is the moment to write the standards for the area you have chosen to audit.

It is important to have written your objectives, because the standards should reflect objectives and philosophy written previously. Standards make explicit the level of quality and they become the bench-marks against which performance is judged.

There are several benefits of setting standards. The first is obvious, and that is monitoring. Monitoring of standards gives professionals the chance to see how well care is delivered and whether standards are being achieved.

Standards may also be used to introduce new knowledge. What better way is there to introduce a new approach to clinical care than to identify and agree, as a professional group, what has to be done and to set the standard to establish the level at which all the staff must perform, when implementing a new aspect of clinical care with consistency throughout the team?

Standards may also be used to identify deficiencies. It may be difficult to achieve a standard because a particular piece of equipment is not available and therefore the outcome cannot be achieved satisfactorily; or it may be that there are insufficient staff, or the wrong skill-mix of staff.

From a professional point of view the next benefit, which is making explicit what we do, may be one of the most important areas in which standards are written. As individuals we know exactly how everyone within our profession works, what we do, what our objectives are, what our aims are and how we achieve good quality patient care. But how much do we know about other professions? How much do we understand about how they work, their professional codes of conduct, how they apply their clinical practice and how it interlinks with our own? Setting standards, particularly multidisciplinary standards, is an opportunity to get together to understand how to work as a team and to set standards that make explicit what we do. Standard setting is important because not only does it make explicit what we do, but it also makes explicit what we need to have in order to undertake that care and what we expect as the outcome; in other words: structure, process and outcome criteria.

2.1 Basic principles of setting standards

The principles and the approach to setting standards are written in detail in Chapter 3, but for the sake of clarity here, I shall review the basic principles of setting standards as part of clinical audit.

- The first principle is that the whole group should agree on the standard. Standards are not set by one person sitting behind closed doors, in an office, setting standards for other people. One of the main benefits of standard setting is that staff are given the opportunity to discuss their approaches to clinical care, the delivery of patient care, how it is done and how it should be done. The resulting standard is the agreed standard about approaches to patient care which leads to consistency and continuity of care for the patient.
- Standards are written by the people who deliver the care, they are not imposed and they are owned by the people who write them. It is essential that standards are written by the people who deliver care, as standards cannot be written by people who are not in the clinical area delivering care on a day-to-day basis. It is also important to mention at this point that standards must be research-based. They must reflect up-to-date, good clinical practice.
- Standards must contain the indicators of quality for a particular service or care group. So it is important to identify the indicators of quality, what makes this service good and then reflect the findings within the standards that are written.
- Standards are valid definitions of quality of care. Standards cannot be valid unless they contain the means of measuring

them, in the form of criteria. The criteria make the standard work, they are the items that are measurable within the standard. These criteria are found in structure, process and outcome. It is important to note that a standard is not a standard unless it *can be* measured, and a standard is not a standard until it *has been* measured and validated.

- It is essential that standards are monitored regularly by the group or from outside the group. What is should be compared with what should be according to the standard, and action should be taken to ensure the gap is closed. It is this last section, the identification of the gaps and taking action to close them, that ensures that standards are achieved. This is perhaps the most essential part of the whole process of setting standards.

3. Agree, implement and monitor change

This principle leads on from the section above: the first step is to monitor the standards and identify current performance. The clinical audit process will identify areas of excellence and also identify areas in need of improvement. At this point, in clinical audit, the ways of improving patient care must be discussed and agreed by the group.

Clinical audit is not something that is taken on by one person, it is achieved by a group of people. This means that the tasks and the workload should be shared among the group and individual people should be made responsible for specific areas of work that have been identified.

4. Communication

Within the organisation in which the clinical audit studies are taking place, there needs to be a communication strategy to publicise the purpose and the outcome of audit so that the results may be shared for the benefit of patients throughout the organisation, and also to prevent duplication of studies. Communication should not be limited purely to the professionals involved in audit but also be extended to patients and their relatives, particularly with issues such as the audit of pain control.

Audits will be multidisciplinary and the outcomes will affect people in a variety of departments who perhaps were not involved in the original audit. Communication should also be aimed at management, at the policy-makers and at those who are accountable for the resources, because without their support identified changes with resource implications may never take place.

Potential Problems

One of the problems that has been identified within the principle of communication is the lack of involvement of management within the clinical audit process. In my experience the involvement of management at the very beginning of the audit is vital and should include presenting them with:

- the objectives for the study
- the area to be audited
- the reason for the audit
- a list of the people who are likely to be involved
- the resources that are likely to be required
- the potential outcome, with the potential changes to practice and potential resource implications all clearly identified.

It is important to gain their support from the beginning, because without this support you may undertake an extremely worthwhile audit, only to find that when the results are discussed the organisation cannot afford to implement the changes. This is very disheartening for everybody involved, as a lot of time and effort has been put into establishing an effective audit with results that require change.

One of the main areas of concern during an audit is confidentiality, as often patients' records, information and data are used to establish the findings within the audit. It is essential that there is a policy on confidentiality and that everyone is clear about what that means, and that all data is anonymous. There may also be a variety of people involved in audit, such as data collection clerks, secretaries, and other people who are not bound by a professional code of conduct, so this issue of confidentiality needs to be addressed and assured.

While undertaking clinical audit, sometimes poor practice involving a particular individual is identified. Prior to the study it is important to establish what the policy and the procedure is in the event of this being discovered. This is one of the areas that causes anxiety to staff. Staff worry that they will be found to be doing something that is either inappropriate or negligent and are concerned that they will be identified and taken to task. The organisation as a whole needs to have a very clear policy on what the procedure is in the event of poor practice being identified.

One of the reasons for setting clearly stated objectives at the start of the study, and also the standards defining the boundaries of the study, is to ensure that the study does not become too large. It is easy to become over-enthusiastic about what you are doing and for the members for the group to say 'wouldn't it be interesting if we looked at this and that', and the 'this' and the 'that' take the group way beyond the original objectives and the boundaries of the study into the realms of a different study. So it is essential to keep a very close eye on the size of the study and ensure it does not become too large.

Another problem with audit is the collection and collation of large amounts of data. Again, the group can get over enthusiastic about the collection of data and forget that at the end of the day somebody has to collate it. It is important to be selective about the data that is required and to ensure that the data collected is essential.

There are two major problems that will lead to a failed audit and there is nothing more depressing than an audit that is definitely beginning to fail! The first of these problems is the lack of understanding by the group about what they are meant to be doing. It is important that they are given very clear guidelines as to:

- what the audit is
- what the objectives are
- what the expected outcomes might be
- what their role is
- how they are expected to perform.

The second problem is the lack of commitment within groups that set up audits. Within groups there may be staff who will say 'why bother', 'what good will it do anyway?'. This lack of commitment needs to be addressed before the audit starts, because people with this attitude will destroy the audit from within, they will devalue it and in the end the audit is likely to fail. As stated above, often this lack of commitment is due to lack of understanding and a fear that they will be identified as not performing. These fears and anxieties need to be overcome by careful training and support throughout the study.

The Eleven Steps to Successful Audit

Having outlined the four principles of audit the next step is to put these principles into practice. The cycle of audit activity which results in a systematic improvement in clinical practice can be described in eleven steps. Figure 16 shows the eleven steps to audit. The text that follows describes each step and how that step leads to the next.

1. Win the support and commitment of colleagues

The first part of this step is to obtain support from management, as discussed earlier in this chapter. Without their support, audit is likely to flounder because of the lack of resource. It is important to reiterate at this point that the involvement of management, through the presentation of clear objectives and the likely implications of the audit, will move the group closer to good communication with the managers. During this first step it is a good idea to establish whether there are any specific resources available for audit. These may be in the form of data collection clerks, information technology systems or even other resources such as particular personnel with expertise or access to previous studies that are closely linked to the proposed audit.

The research undertaken at the beginning of this study, which looks at the mission statement and the objectives of the organisation followed by your own philosophy and objectives,

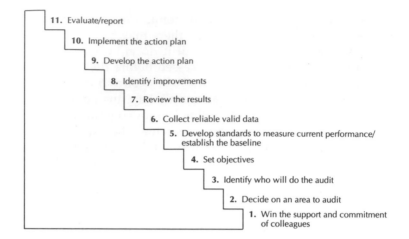

11. Evaluate/report

10. Implement the action plan

9. Develop the action plan

8. Identify improvements

7. Review the results

6. Collect reliable valid data

5. Develop standards to measure current performance/establish the baseline

4. Set objectives

3. Identify who will do the audit

2. Decide on an area to audit

1. Win the support and commitment of colleagues

Figure 16   The eleven steps to audit

will be key in demonstrating how your audit will fit in to the quality assurance strategy for the whole organisation. If this is the case, then the audit is more likely to get support from management.

2. Decide on an area to audit

If you already have standards which are being monitored and have identified an area where it is felt that performance could be improved, then the selection of the area to audit is quite logical, because it follows from the areas measured through your standards. If, on the other hand, there has been no standard setting activity, standards have not been monitored and there are no particular areas that need to be audited, then the following questions might help with the decision.

- Review areas of clinical care and ask: why do staff do it *that* way? Then identify ways that it might be done and ask why don't staff do it this way?
- Are there delays in the provision of care? If so why do these delays occur and what can be done to improve the timing of provision of care?
- Discuss with colleagues whether or not patients have unnecessary complications. If they do, what can be done about

it? In what specific areas do these complications occur?
- Discuss whether equipment is always used correctly and if not, what can be done about it?
- Are the most suitably qualified people delivering the care? Who is doing what, who should be doing what?
- A key area to address is whether or not clinical practice is safe. If not, why not and how can it be improved?
- Finally, would a change in resources improve the quality of care? What resources are available at present, what resources are required and where are the gaps?

Areas for audit may also include areas of clinical care that are high volume, high risk or high cost. The area selected may stem from a complaint or a critical incident. Or there may be outside pressures such as a purchaser requirement, a Health of the Nation target, the Patient's Charter, an area of care or concern raised by the Community Health Council or any other outside body.

3. Identify who will do the audit

The group to conduct the audit will probably arise quite naturally from the chosen area in which the audit is being undertaken, whether it be a ward, department, a whole hospital, the patient's home or community. As mentioned above under the topic of resources, there may be key people available who will affect the choice or make up the group. There may be several groups of people working at various levels of the organisation. It may be important to involve some of the managers with the audit to ensure that both sides of the clinical audit are taken into account, that is, clinical care and the management of that care.

In the UK, at present, some clinical audits are undertaken by uniprofessional groups but clinical audit of patient care should be a multidisciplinary team approach where everybody who has a part to play in patient care is involved. It is very difficult to isolate one group of professionals delivering patient care without taking into account how the other professionals impact upon the care that has been given.

The initial activities within this third step provide a good opportunity to set up some workshops and seminars to get everybody started, to make sure they are well informed and have a clear understanding so that they may participate totally without feeling unsure of themselves.

Having identified the *scope* of the audit, decide how much *time* should be spent on the audit. The staff who are involved in clinical audit already have a heavy professional work load, are working hard delivering patient care and this activity comes as an extra activity. So be realistic about how much time is required and how much time can be given to deliver a successful audit. Also at this point, it is important to consider what the audit will require apart from time. Will it require, for example:

● information technology?
● the development of data collection forms?
● secretarial support?

3.1 Evidence base

Clinical audit must be evidence based, in other words based on recognised research evidence that is proven to be effective or expert clinical judgement. This will involve a literature search to establish current research findings, through a computer search. However, many audit topics deal with local issues for which the literature may provide only evidence that is of superficial relevance. In this case it is even more important to develop local standards and criteria through discussion with the relevant stakeholders.

An evidence base may also be provided through existing protocols, national initiatives, professional consensus, peer group consensus.

4. Set the objectives for the audit

The objectives should be set and agreed by the audit group. Objectives must be measurable and achievable and in line with the strategy and objectives for the audit programme and the organisation as a whole, as set out in the business plan and the quality assurance plan.

5. Develop standards to measure current performance

If there are no standards, or if existing standards have not been monitored, then this is the moment to agree, write and set the standards specifically for the audit that you have in mind.

Every standard should be broken down into measurable elements that will indicate whether or not it is being met. These are known as *audit indicators* or *audit criteria*. The audit indicators or audit criteria are the criteria that have been established within the structure, process and outcome criteria of the standard. (For more information on standard setting see Chapter 3.) The audit indicators are the foundations around which to collect data.

Establishing the baseline or identifying the level of current practice may also be achieved though a comparison with other centres, through clinical judgement or the assessment of current practice through direct observation.

6. Collect the data

There are already numerous potential sources from which to gather relevant data without gathering new data of your own. The patient or client record is a key area. The care plans developed by nurses and by other professionals also contain information that may be relevant to the particular audit. The audit may require a review of the Complaints Reports, so establish who is responsible for the complaints received from patients and relatives and then talk to them and establish if there have been any complaints relating to the area of the selected audit. Another area that may be relevant to the audit is the accident reports indicating numbers of patient falls or staff incidents.

There is an enormous amount of data to be gathered from the Korner-based data. This data will give you information on length of stay, cases per consultant and bed occupancy. So if this information is relevant to the audit, make arrangements to gather it from the finance department or the information technology department or whichever department it is that holds it. If in doubt as to where this data is held, then ask at the library: the staff will probably be able to tell you where you can obtain it.

The audit may require new sources of information to be developed. It is important to try to keep this information down to what is essential. It is also important to use forms that are already in existence to save the staff having to learn how new forms are to be filled in. This also saves money that might be spent on the reproduction of numerous new forms. So look at existing forms and see if these can be used. If they are not exactly what you need, then it may be possible to modify them. If not, you will need to develop a new form. Make sure when the audit form is developed that it is clear and easy to understand and quick to complete. Again, remember this is something people are undertaking in addition to their usual work load. If there are several audits in progress at one time, then staff will be spending a disproportionate amount of time completing audit data collection forms.

It may be necessary to conduct interviews with patients, clients or other service users. If the use of interviewing is to be one of the areas for collecting data, then make sure that the key questions to be asked are written down in an unambiguous fashion, so that all the interviewers ask the same questions. This will facilitate the collection of the data. It may be necessary to create a special audit questionnaire, in which case the information on developing questionnaires in Chapter 3 may be helpful. In the majority of clinical audit studies the staff are involved in observing and recording patient information and data. If this is the case, then the forms on which they record data must be clearly designed, easy to understand and quick to complete. Remember that it is in these areas that there may be problems with confidentiality, so ensure that whatever is developed is in line with the hospital's policy on confidentiality.

For the chosen topic to be audited decide which data are essential to the audit answer the following questions:

● What are the purposes of the data?
● What data items are required?
● What are the sources of the data?

Only collect essential data that will support each stage of the audit cycle. To confirm the problem, identify the underlying cause of the problem, provide evidence for the need for change, and evaluate the changes made.

6.1 Sample size

You will need to give some thought to the sample size of data to be collected. The sample used must be large enough to meet the objectives of the audit but not so large that unnecessary time is spent collecting and collating data that are not required or has no purpose. The skills of a statistician may be helpful in making an accurate decision but experience and clinical judgement will tell you what is a reasonable sample size.

6.2 Pilot the data collection systems

Pilot all aspects of data collection to ensure that the data collected is accurate, reliable, ethical and valid. Check that all data collection forms result in the collection of data that meets the purpose as intended, are non ambiguous and straightforward to use.

7. Review the results

Once everybody has collected all the data required, the next step is the analysis. The analysis of data can take a great deal of time and so it is essential to be sure the data collected was really required and essential and no more. Taking each indicator in turn, quantify the degree to which the standards have been met and identify areas where the service delivered has not conformed to the standards set. This needs to be clearly documented as the group collate and analyse the data.

During this process the group may discover that one indicator has a significantly lower rate of achievement than the others, or there is a pattern of failure which is emerging which indicates a need for a specific remedy. It is important to note down the indicators and the way that the study is actually progressing and to discuss them at regular meetings of the whole group, so that everyone is clear about how the study is going.

8. Identify improvements

Through analysis of the data and peer group discussion identify improvements to be made, if these are necessary.

9. Develop an action plan

The action plan should identify how the group intends to rectify any problems that the audit has identified. This action plan should specify the following:

- the improvement to be achieved
- the actions that need to be taken
- the resources (if any) that are needed
- how their achievement can be measured
- the timescale by which improvements should be achieved
- who is responsible.

One method of exploring possible solutions is for the group to focus on one particular problem through brainstorming, or by using a mock solution in a systematic way. It is essential that ideas are explored on paper or within the group prior to using them with direct patient care. If the outcome of the audit indicates a change in the delivery of patient care it is essential that those changes are piloted and the results monitored prior to implementation on a larger scale.

10. Implement the action plan

Once the action plan has been drawn up and named people have been identified to co-ordinate certain aspects of the initiative, then it is essential that the new strategy is put into effect. Any changes should reflect the results of the monitoring process and these may have to be modified again after a further period of evaluation. This should not necessarily be seen as the end result, as there may need to be further changes to ensure that the delivery of care has been improved to the extent which was initially predicted.

11. Evaluate and report

Once the group is confident that the standards are now firmly in place, that changes have been identified and those changes when measured assure the group that the quality of care has been improved and can be sustained, then the audit report can prepared for all those involved in the service and for management.

General Points

Throughout the process of clinical audit it is essential that key people within each area are made responsible for keeping the whole group informed of what is happening, how the audit is progressing, and ensuring that the group meets to discuss findings, problems and the way forward. Key people from within each audit would benefit from spending some time on networking with other people working with other audits: this will help prevent duplication, overlap, repetition and replications of studies.

After an audit it is interesting to note that staff are often highly encouraged about the process, as it gives them a feeling of autonomy over their professional practice. There is a sense of achievement that they have the ability and the wherewithal to make changes to improve patient care. They are usually inspired to go on the next audit, to take the next area and to try to improve things for their patients.

Setting up the first audit is the most difficult and also the most crucial. If an audit has been set up well, has been thought through, with a clear idea of what the outcome might be, then the audit is often successful. Poor preparation for audit, with unclear objectives, poorly set standards that are not monitorable or measurable, and a vague idea of what the outcome might be, will often lead to an audit that falls apart half way through. This does not inspire people to go on to audit further areas. In fact it has the opposite effect and it makes them feel 'why bother'.

Sometimes the audit is not successful and after the data collection and the implementation of change the standard is still not achieved. This means that there needs to be further change in practice in specific areas. The group needs to go back and look at the data it collected, the documentation that it reviewed and in general review the notes made on the audit as it progressed, and try to identify where the gaps were, what should have been reviewed and was not reviewed. The other area that needs to be reviewed when an audit is unsuccessful is: how well did staff understand their role in the audit? Was there room for further educational sessions for the staff? Were the staff committed to the principle of audit or did their lack of commitment contribute to the failure of the audit?

Whatever the outcome, there will definitely be a greater understanding of the area of work the group has undertaken, and greater appreciation of other people's roles and responsibilities and how staff work as a team. There is nearly always a renewed commitment to professional competence and in most cases the competence breeds confidence.

Finally, the result of all this work is development of explicit quality indicators and an improvement in patient care, which after all is what it is all about.

Guidelines for Success

In this section I have summarised the elements which I believe lead to a successful audit.

Commitment
- Commitment to the study
- Group of staff who are keen to be involved

Scale of the study
- Start with a small study.
- Be clear about the scope of the study.

Learn – key elements
- Handling the data
- Getting information from outside about current practice
- Drawing up checklists
- Devising ways of communicating
- Developing resources

Decisions to be made
- How is the audit to be carried out?
- What should be looked at?
- How should it be studied?
- What should be done with the results?

Rules for success
- Look at topics that are relevant to the group's work.
- Ensure professional groups maintain responsibility for their own practice.
- Be clear about policies, procedures and confidentiality.
- Ensure the study is not too time-consuming.

Examples of areas for clinical audit might include:

- patient information on diagnosis, treatment/care, follow up care
- post operative wound infections
- prevalence of pressure sores
- immunisation uptake and health promotion
- staffing numbers and skill-mix including doctors, nurses, therapists, clerical staff, support staff
- the security of records
- discharge of patients and follow-up care
- lifting and moving of patients
- confidentiality
- communication with staff
- waiting times and waiting lists.

Below is an example of a multidisciplinary standard set for the discharge of patients which has been selected as an area to audit as the standards have not been achieved in specific areas.

The main problem areas are as follows:

Example 1

- The patients were not given any indication of their predicted length of stay on admission.
- The patients were not told they were going home until the day before, or even, on one or two occasions, on the day of discharge.
- An area of concern highlighted by patients was that they felt they were not given enough information about how they should care for themselves at home. This information was often verbal and not backed up with anything in writing.

Standard statement: Every patient's discharge plan is commenced on admission, completed 24 hours prior to discharge and meets his or her identified needs to ensure continuity of care.

Structure criteria:
- Structured discharge plan
- Staff skills and knowledge

→

- Discharge check list
- Written information concerning specific patient care at home

Process criteria:
- On admission the doctor advises the patient or relatives on the predicted length of stay.
- The professional team assess the patient's needs prior to discharge (as an on-going process).
- A discharge plan is developed from admission.
- The discharge plan is discussed with the patient or relatives.
- Home care is discussed with the patient or relatives.
- The discharge plan is completed 24 hours prior to discharge.
- The discharge checklist is completed prior to discharge.

Outcome criteria:
- There is documented evidence that:

	YES	NO
— the discharge was commenced on admission	☐	☐
— the discharge plan was updated as the patient's stay progressed	☐	☐
— the patient's needs were assessed	☐	☐
— the discharge plan was completed	☐	☐
— the discharge plan was completed at least 24 hours prior to discharge	☐	☐
— the discharge checklist was completed.	☐	☐

- The patient or relatives can state that:

	YES	NO
— he or she was given an indication of the predicted length of stay on admission to hospital	☐	☐
— the discharge plan was planned with him or her	☐	☐
— the plan met their needs	☐	☐
— he or she was given verbal information concerning his or her care at home	☐	☐
— he or she was given written information concerning his or her care at home.	☐	☐

Audit indicators from criteria in the standards:
- Review the patient's medical, nursing or therapy records for evidence of:
  - doctor's advice to patient concerning predicted length of stay on admission
  - the professional team assessment of the patient's needs prior to discharge
  - the discharge plan and its continued development over the patient's stay
  - discussions with relatives and patients about care at home.

- Collect length of stay data
- Collect readmission data

→

- Monitor the discharge plan through a checklist.
  This check list requires a 'yes' or 'no' answer to each
  of the following.   YES   NO
  — Discharge planning commenced on admission.   ☐   ☐
  — Services required at home were identified.   ☐ . ☐
  — Services were organised.   ☐   ☐
  — Services were organised at least 24 hours prior to
    discharge.   ☐   ☐
  — Discharge plan was completed.   ☐   ☐
  — Discharge plan was completed at least 24 hours
    prior to discharge.   ☐   ☐
  — Discharge checklist was completed prior to
    discharge.   ☐   ☐

- Ask questions through interviews with patients
  and relatives.   YES   NO
  — Were you given an indication of how long you
    would be in hospital?   ☐   ☐
  — Was the discharge plan discussed with you?   ☐   ☐
  — What is the plan for your discharge?   ☐   ☐
  — When were you told you were going home?   ☐   ☐
  — Did the plan meet your needs?   ☐   ☐
  — Did someone explain how you were to care for
    yourself at home?   ☐   ☐
  — Were you given any written information about how
    to care for yourself at home?   ☐   ☐

Exercise 4

- Identify the topic on which you have decided to conduct an audit.
- Identify who would be involved in the audit.
- Identify the evidence base.
- Set the objectives for the audit.
- Identify the standard which supports the audit.
- Identify the audit indicators from within the criteria from the standard.
- List the audit indicators and identify how you will monitor each indicator.
- Identify the data to be collected.
- Identify what resources would be required.
- Try to predict the outcome of the audit.

Further Reading

Chase, R. L. (ed.) *TQM* (New York: IFS Publications).

Crombie, I. K., H. T. O. Davies, S. C. S. Abraham, C. du V. Florey, *The Audit Handbook – Improving Health Care through Clinical Audit* (Chichester: John Wiley & Sons, 1993).

DoH, *Working for Patients* (London: HMSO, 1990).

DoH, *Meeting and improving standards in healthcare; a policy document on the development of clinical audit*, EL(93)59 (Heywood: Department of Health, 1993).

DoSS *Management's Arrangement for the Reorganised NHS* (London: HMSO, 1972).

Fitzpatrick, R., Surveys of patient satisfaction: 11 Designing a questionnaire and conducting a survey, *British Medical Journal;* 1991 302: 1129–32.

Getting Ahead with Clinical Audit: a Facilitator's Guide published by the NHS Training Directorate and the NHSE, 1994).

Hendrick, T. E., *PreJIT/TQC. Audit: First Step of the Journey* (1988).

Hopkins, A., *Measuring the quality of medical care* (London Royal College of Physicians, 1990).

Jones, S., 'Medical Audit (Surgery)', *The International Journal of Health Care and Quality Assurance* (1990).

Koch, Dr. Hugh *Total Quality Management in Health Care* (Longman, 1981).

Kogan, M. and S. Redfern, *Making use of clinical audit* (Buckingham: Open University Press, 1995).

Lewis, N., 'Nursing Audit', *International Journal of Health Care and Quality Assurance.* Feb 1919.

Mason, A., *Enabling Clinical Work in the South West* (Bristol: SWHRA, 1990).

NHSME, *Nursing Care Audit* (Labor: HMSO).

RCP, *Medical Audit: A first report* (London, 1989).

Shaw, C., *Medical Audit Hospital Handbook* (King's Fund Centre, 1989).

South Western Regional Health Authority, SWRHA, *Regional Approach to Medical Audit* (Bristol: SWRHA, 1989).

Walshe, K. and J. Bennett, *Guidelines on medical audit and confidentiality* (Brighton Health Authority/South East Thames Regional Health Authority, 1991).

Chapter 5   Clinical Protocols

Background

The principle of clinical protocols leads on naturally from the preceding chapters on standards and audit. The approach that I am about to describe derives from work undertaken on behalf of Price Waterhouse with St James' Hospital in Leeds on the development of clinical protocols. A protocol is a plan giving details of steps that will be followed.

This particular clinical protocol is a combination of a patient tracking system, anticipated recovery pathways, standards and workload. The system allows you to track the progress of patient care from referral from the GP through the hospital, on to discharge and then back to the community.

An Example of a Clinical Protocol

In our example (Figure 17) there are four main columns, which relate to *structure*, *process*, *outcome* and *monitoring* or *measurement*. The first column, 'Professional Input', looks at who is responsible for the particular aspect of care, what grade of staff, and how long it will take them to undertake a particular task. This column is directly linked to the care profile (process) in the third column demonstrating what that professional must do in order to achieve the quality indicator (or outcome) in the next column.

This is an expected outcome for all patients to achieve within a time limit. In the final column there are ways of monitoring this and whether the outcome has been achieved or not. If the

Figure 17 Example of a first time hip replacement (from St James' Hospital, Leeds, 1993)

St James' Hospital
TREATMENT PROFILE – HIP REPLACEMENT (1ST TIME)

Professional input	In-patient Day	Care profile	Quality indicator	Measurement
		GP		
		Referral letter to consultant		
Consultant 10 mins		*Consultant sorts referral letters into urgency*	Letter to GP within *...days of receipt of referral letter	Business Manager Ongoing
		letter to GP	Patient receives OPD appointment holding letter to patient received within *... days	Report to Clinical Director monthly report to Trust Board 6 monthly
Consultant 10 mins		*Consultant Clinic OPD*		
		– Patient seen by consultant – X-Ray at same appointment, or – X-Ray arranged by GP – Report + X-Ray seen at clinic	Routine appointments within *... weeks letter includes: Named surgeon/clinic telephone number extension to contact map of site, clinic/department	
		To GP		
		No need for surgery		Patient satisfaction
		May need surgery in the future		
		Patient requires surgery		
		Investigation Bloods taken	OPD staff are helpful and courteous	Clinical Audit
		Results to notes and GP	Tests and investigations as appropriate	Clinical Audit
		GP Treats abnormalities		

* This will be filled in according to the local standard

Professional input	In-patient Day	Care profile	Quality indicator	Measurement
Administrative staff _10_ mins		Waiting list Patient name in suspension pending GP treatment → Patient added to Acute waiting list	Common waiting list for hips and knees in Chronological order Patient not necessarily operated on by original consultant unless specifically requested	Business manager ongoing, report to Clinical Director monthly Report to Trust Board 6 monthly
SHO 20 mins Anaesthetist 20 mins Home visit 60 mins Clinic 15 mins		Patient's on the Acute waiting list *Pre-admission Clinic* 2 weeks pr or to surgery Assess fitness for surgery *Pre-admission visit from OT* Home visit — Clinic	Waiting list for surgery * . . . weeks Pre-admission clinic held once per week – at present only serves waiting list initiative patients – plans to expand to all patients Every patient assessed – the OT prior to surgery	Business Manager patient satisfaction Clinical audit
	Day 1	*Pre-admission Routine* *Admission* Same day — 1 day prior to surgery	Pre-admission information includes: Date of admission; Ward; Consultant; PT information handbook Appropriate staff available Bed available Facilities are clean, comfortable and welcoming	Business Manager ongoing Manpower monitoring Business Manager Audit health and safety Patient satisfaction

* This will be filled in according to the local standard

St James' Hospital
TREATMENT PROFILE – HIP REPLACEMENT (1ST TIME)

Professional input	In-patient Day	Care profile	Quality indicator	Measurement
RGN 30 mins	Day 1	*Admission Routine* *Admitted by nursing staff* (Nursing assessment (Draw up plan of care (Urinalysis (Base line observations (Weight (Measured for TD stockings	Patient orientated to ward within 10 mins of arrival Assessment completed within 2 hours of patient's arrival Care is planned with patients and documented within 2 hours of arrival Discharge planning begins on admission	Ongoing Monitoring of standards by peer review Results to clinical director annually
SHO: Patient admitted direct to ward – 20 mins		Seen by SHO Patient admitted via Pre-admission Clinic Patient admitted Direct to ward	Medical assessment Clerking within 1 hour of arrival	Clinical audit
SHO: Patient admitted via Pre-admission Clinic – 10 mins		Brief check Assessed and clerked Clerked Consent form signed Consent form signed	Informed consent obtained	Monitor standard
Anaesthetist:		Seen by Anaesthetist	Anaesthetic assessment prior to premedication	Clinical audit
Patient admitted direct to ward – 20 mins		Patient admitted via Pre–admission Patient admitted Clinic – assess fitness Direct to ward for surgery		
Patient admitted via Pre-admission Clinic – 10 mins		Complete physical Examination		

98

Professional input	In-patient Day	Care profile	Quality indicator	Measurement
SHO 10 mins	Day 1 continued	*Tests and investigations* - - - - - - - - - - Bloods for groups as required – X-Ray chest - ECG Commence anticoagillant therapy - - - - - - for 10 days – commencing 12 hours prior to surgery – as soon as possible for patients admitted same day surgery	- - - - Tests and investigations as appropriate - - - Prevention of DVT	Clinical audit Clinical audit
RGN Theatre nurse 20 mins		*Pre-theatre visit by theatre staff* - - - - - - - Patient meets theatre nurse who will receive him or her into Anaesthetic room Nurse discusses care patient will receive in theatre	- - - Patient has a named nurse to greet him/her Patient has a clear idea of theatre routine	Patient satisfaction
Nurse any level 20 mins	Day 2	Patient fasting regime established		
		Day of operation		
RGN 10 mins Other nurse 10 mins		Routine preparation for theatre all consultants same regime	Patient received emotional and physical support in accordance with hospital guidelines Information to patient and relatives – informed consent re-confirmed prior to premedication – Pre operative check – List completed	Monitoring of standards Results to Clinical Director annually Patient satisfaction
RGN 10 mins		Premedication		
RGN 3rd year student 10 mins Porters × 2 total = 40 mins		Final pre-operating check Escort to theatre		Patient satisfaction

St James' Hospital
TREATMENT PROFILE – HIP REPLACEMENT (1ST TIME)

Professional input	In-patient Day	Care profile	Quality indicator	Measurement
RGN 25 mins	Day 2 Continued	*Theatre – Anaesthetic room* Received by named nurse Pre-operative check list Completed by receiving nurse	Patient received in theatre by nurse who visited patient on ward	Patient satisfaction
Consultant 20 mins Anaesthetic 25 mins		Patient seen by surgeon Consultant surgeon stays with patient until anaesthetised Checks: Correct patient Correct surgery Correct medical records Correct X-Rays	Correct patient Correct surgical intervention Preparation for theatre completed	Monitor standards
Consultant 1 hr 30 mins Sen Reg/Reg 1 hr 30 mins Anaesthetist 1 hr 40 mins Consultant 10 mins RGN × 3 total 30 mins		*Theatre – Surgery* Surgical intervention Blood transfusion × 3 units Anaesthetic – wake up Prior to move to recovery Clean up theatre for next case	Surgical intervention completed Patient conscious Safely recovered Theatre clean for next patient	Clinical audit Clinical audit Monitor standards Report to clinical director annually
Anaesthetic 5 mins RGN 30 mins		*Recovery room* Patient returned to consciousness	Patient responds to name Patient conscious	
RGN 10 mins		*Patient returned to Ward* Nurse from ward collects patient Receives report on: Drains Stitches/clips Medicines given and IV infusion regime	Continuity of care between theatre and ward Patient escorted in a dignified manner	Monitor standards: Reports to clinical director annually

100

Professional input	In-patient Day	Care profile	Quality indicator	Measurement
RGN 20 mins 1 other nurse 20 mins Porters 40 mins	Day 2 Continued	*Patient escorted back to ward* Patient made comfortable Positioning Observations IV checked Drains and dressings	Patient transferred safely back toward continuity of care	Monitor standards Results to clinical director annually
RGN 15 mins 1 other nurse 15 mins RGN 180 mins SHO 10 mins Senior Reg 5 mins Nurses 60 mins		*Post-operative care – immediate* Pain control 1 hourly observations for 6 hours 2 hourly observations for 4 hours 4 hourly observations for 48 hours Post op visit by SHO, Senior Reg Total patient care	Pain is controlled to patient's satisfaction Patient observed continuously Patient seen by doctor post operatively	Clinical unit

Nurses 4 hrs = 8 hrs
per shift
SHO × 10 mins
Nurses × 20 mins
Nurse escort RGN 60 mins
SHO 10 mins
Senior Reg 5–10 mins
Physiotherapy 20–25 mins
OT 20 mins
	Day 3	*1st post-operative day*
		Total patient care
		Post op bloods
		Post op X-Ray in X-Ray dept
		SHO visit
		Senior Registrar visit
		Mobilise:
		    Physiotherapy
		    OT – talk and advise
		    Nursing staff
		
		4-hourly observations
			Appropriate total care recorded in records
			Monitoring of patient post operative care
			
			Patient is seen by a doctor daily and medical notes updated daily
			Patient mobilising
				Ongoing peer review
				
				Clinical audit

St James' Hospital
TREATMENT PROFILE – HIP REPLACEMENT (1ST TIME)

Professional input	In-patient Day	Care profile	Quality indicator	Measurement
2 nurses – 4 hours = 8 hours per shift	Day 4	*2nd post-operative day* Total patient care Mobilisation 4-hourly observations IV Discontinued Drains out	Appropriate total care recorded in records Mobilising patient	Ongoing peer review
Physiotherapy 25 mins OT 20 mins SHO 15 mins Senior Reg 10 mins		Physiotherapy OT – Talk and Advise visit by SHO Senior Registrar →	Mobilising patient Patient seen daily by a doctor and medical notes updated daily	Ongoing peer review Clinical audit
2 nurses 4 hours = 8 hours per shift Physiotherapy 60 mins	Day 5	*3rd post-operative day* Total patient care Mobilisation 6-hourly observations	Appropriate total care recorded in records Mobilising patient	Ongoing peer review Ongoing peer review
OT 90 mins SHO 90 mins Senior Reg 10 mins Consultant 5 mins		Physiotherapy OT Visit by SHO Senior Registrar Consultant (ward round) →	Patients seen daily by a doctor and medical notes updated daily	Clinical audit
Nurses 2 hours = 4 hours per shift	Day 6	*4th post-operative day* Assist patient with all aspects of care Mobilisation 6-hourly observations	Appropriate care recorded in records	Ongoing peer review
Physiotherapy 90 mins OT 90 mins SHO 15 mins Senior Reg 10 mins		Physiotherapy OT Visit by SHO Senior Registrar →	Mobilising patient Patient seen daily by a doctor and medical notes updated daily	Ongoing peer review Clinical audit

Professional input	In-patient Day	Care profile	Quality indicator	Measurement
2 nurses – 4 hours = 8 hours per shift	Day 7	*5th post-operative day* Assist patient with all aspects of care	Appropriate care Recorded in records	Ongoing peer review
Physiotherapy 60 mins OT 90 mins SHO 15 mins Senior Reg 10 mins		Mobilisation BD observations Physiotherapy OT – include kitchen assessment as required Visit by SHO Senior Registrar	Mobilising patient rehabilitation Patient seen daily by a doctor and medical notes updated daily	Ongoing peer review Clinical audit
Nurses 45 mins per shift	Day 8	*6th post-operative day* Assist patient with all aspects of care Mobilisation BD observations	Appropriate care received in records	Ongoing peer review
Physiotherapy 45 mins OT 15 mins SHO 15 mins Senior Reg 10 mins		Physiotherapy OT Visit by SHO Senior Registrar	Mobilising and rehabilitating patient Patient seen daily by a doctor and medical records updated daily	Ongoing peer review Clinical audit
		Discharge plan review	Ongoing plan for discharge with patient	Monitor standard report to Clinical Director annually

St James' Hospital
TREATMENT PROFILE – HIP REPLACEMENT (1ST TIME)

Professional input	In-patient Day	Care profile	Quality indicator	Measurement
Same as 6th post-operative day	Day 9	*7th post-operative day* Same as 6th post-operative day	Same as 6th post-operative day	Same as 6th post-operative day
RGN nursing 20 mins per shift	Day 10	*8th post-operative day* Assist patient with care as required Daily observations Clips/stitches out Dressing Mobilisation	Appropriate care recorded in records	Ongoing peer review
Physiotherapy 30 mins OT 30 mins SHO 10 mins Senior Reg 5 mins Consultant 5 mins		Physiotherapy OT Visit by SHO Senior Registrar Consultant (ward round)	Mobilisation and rehabilitation Patient seen daily by a doctor and medical records updated daily	Ongoing peer review Clinical audit
RGN 20 mins per shift Ward clerk 30 mins Physiotherapy 10 mins OT 10 mins SHO 5 mins Senior Reg 5 mins	Day 11	*9th post-operative day* Day prior to discharge Daily observations Final discharge arrangements Co-ordination of discharge Patient self-caring	Appropriate care recorded in records Discharge plan recorded	Ongoing peer review Monitoring of standards report to Clinical Director annually
		Physiotherapy OT Visit by SHO Senior Registrar	Mobilisation and rehabilitation Patient seen daily by doctor and medical records updated daily	Ongoing peer review Clinical audit
		Discharged planned		

104

Professional input	In-patient Day	Care profile	Quality indicator	Measurement
Senior Reg 10 mins RGN 10 mins	Day 12	*10th post-operative day* Discharged by Senior Registrar Nurse co-ordinates discharge Complete discharge plan Check list	Patient discharged with all services arranged as assessed	Monitoring standards Patient satisfaction survey
			Community carers informed at least 2 days prior to discharge	Monitor standards
			Co-ordination and continuity is achieved by named person	Audit formal discharge plans
		Patient takes written information concerning care Patient discharged home	Patient and carers involved in discharge plans	Patient satisfaction survey
Secretary 15 mins		Outpatient Recall 1 visit 6–12 weeks · With community care · Without community care · With revisits for therapy	2 discharge letters: – typed day of / day after discharge – sent to/faxed GP	Random samples – monitor records – ask patient/relative – ask GP

105

outcome is not achieved, then the negative outcome is investigated and an action plan developed to resolve the problem.

The protocol was written by the whole team of staff caring for a patient who received a first hip replacement. The protocol reflects what happens in a specific clinical situation and may differ from one hospital to another, depending on local practice.

Development of a Clinical Protocol

When this study began in Leeds it was important that the whole group gathered together, with representatives from all members of staff who had input in to the process of care for a patient who was having a hip replacement for the first time. If possible, it is advantageous to include the GPs and community staff. This is not always possible due to time constraints and if this is the case then a draft copy of the protocol should be sent to the GPs and to representatives of the community staff to gain their comments, approval and any additional points to be added to the protocol.

It is important to discuss the protocol with the community staff, with particular reference to areas where there are time limits for GP action and expected responses from people within the community. The group then discuss the progress of the patient's care from the GP, including time limits, identifying who should be responsible for various aspects of care and estimating how long it will take.

The clinical protocol covers each day and every day of the patient's stay through to discharge. The discussions within the group often uncover areas where there is duplication of activity or where it is preferable for one professional to undertake responsibility for particular aspects of care where in the past there has been more than one professional group involved. During discussions the group may also uncover areas of poor or weak practice which need to be corrected.

It is important to identify, through the outcome of each process of care, what you expect the patient to achieve at this particular time. It is also relevant to discuss what might occur if the patient does not respond to the outcome as expected, for example: a patient who responds badly to the anaesthetic, has breathing difficulties and is required to be transferred to intensive care, rather than transferred directly back to the ward. This loop should be incorporated within the 'possible course' for a patient undergoing surgery.

The benefits of working through a clinical protocol

The benefits of working through a clinical protocol are various, including:

- greater understanding by all members of the Health Care Team as to what each person actually does
- knowing what outcomes are expected
- knowing the time limits as to when outcomes are expected.
- helps staff to think about patient care from a team perspective instead of each profession looking only at the particular area of care for which they are responsible.
- reduces the amount of duplication.
- reduces contradiction of care and leads to greater continuity. For example: a patient is being rehabilitated; the physiotherapists have spent the morning walking him up and down the ward, but at lunchtime, the nurses help him into a wheelchair and wheel him to the table. There is a contradiction in terms of rehabilitation: if it is to be true rehabilitation the nurses should continue the activity by walking the patient to the table.

The professional input column is particularly interesting because it identifies not only who should undertake the care but also how long it takes to deliver the care or treatment. This enables the structure to be costed more accurately in terms of the amount of time spent by professionals, of different grades, in caring for patients. When added to the cost of the equipment and other ongoing costs, this will give a more accurate cost per case than perhaps has been achieved previously.

The column where the outcome is set ensures there is ongoing monitoring of patient response to care rather than monitoring that occurs either just before the patient goes home or on an *ad hoc* or retrospective basis. This ongoing evaluation and monitoring of care will improve the quality of care for patients, using this particular approach.

The Goals of Clinical Protocols

- To promote collaborative practice, co-ordination and continuity of care.
- To direct the contributions of all the health care team towards the achievement of patient outcome.
- To facilitate the achievement of expected patient outcome.
- To facilitate timely discharge within an appropriate length of stay, which is pre-stated.
- To promote appropriate and/or reduce utilisation of resources.
- To promote the working of the Health Care Team together.
- To promote working relationships, not only with the immediate health care team, but also with the community.

This system takes a considerable amount of time to set up but once in place it ensures patients receive greater continuity of care.

Exercise 5

- Identify an area about which you would like to write a clinical protocol.
- Get together with a multidisciplinary group of professionals, identify and track the patient's progress, ensuring that you list: what you need, who you need, how long it will take, what must be done, the expected outcome and how you are going to monitor it.
- Track it right across the entire patient's day, ensuring that you leave nothing out.

Further Reading

American Nurses' Association, The, *Case Management: a challenge for Nurses* (Kansas City, MO: ANA, 1988).

Baker, F. and R. Weiss, 'The nature of case manager support', *Hospital Community Psychiatry*, **35**(9) 925–8.

Berenson, R., 'A physician's prospective on case management', *Business and Health*, **3**(7) 2225.

Zell, D. A. Comeau and K. Zander, 'Nurses' case management, managed care via the nursing case management model', NLN Publication, December 1987, **20**(219) 253–64.

Zander, K., 'Why managed care works', *Definition*, **3**(4) 1–3.

Chapter 6 Monitoring of Providers by Purchasers

The previous chapters of this book have, in the main, described quality assurance approaches that are relevant to the providers of health care. The role of the purchaser in assuring that patients and their relatives receive good quality care is essential.

The guidance for contracting entitled *Operational Principles*[1] stated the importance of quality: 'The contractual process should be directed to improving the quality of services provided and not to efficiency and cost effectiveness alone'. This statement reinforces the principle that providers of care will be competing on quality as well as price.

The six dimensions of quality identified by Maxwell[2] may be used as a simple framework for the contracting process. They are:

- appropriateness
- accessibility
- acceptability
- efficiency
- effectiveness
- equity.

These include clinical and non-clinical aspects of quality. Any service considered to be of good quality would achieve a good standard in each of the six dimensions.

Staff working within a provider unit should have access to the contracts and service specifications that are relevant to the area in which they work, to ensure that they are clear about the requirements of the contract. The format and content of contracts will vary, but the following example will give some

111

idea of what the contract and service specification might contain. The contract will have:

- **A service specification** – within this document will be the priority short-term objectives. These may be broken down into
  — the aims of the service
  — the priority short-term objectives
  — the targets.
- **A schedule of services** – which may include the schedule of when various aspects of the service occur, the location of the service, the availability of the service and an indicative volume of the service/total contacts.

Example 1

A contract for the Health Visiting Service:

Schedule of services:
10–14 day visit

Location:
Home

Availability:
All mothers and babies on the 10/14 day after birth

Indicative volume/Total contacts:
92

The quality aspect of the contract may contain various sections, as described below, using health visiting as an example.

Example 2

Strategic themes:
The provision of a service which is integrated within the Primary Health Care Team

General quality statements:
- Health visitors shall make at least one contact with all ante-natal mothers in the 'at risk' category, and will visit at home if appropriate.
- All children will have developmental checks undertaken by the health visitor at the ages of 7–9 months, 18 months and $3\frac{1}{2}$ years.

➤

> *Monitoring quality:*
> This outlines the agreed quality assurance monitoring programme.
>
> *Developments:*
> This area would include current or new initiatives based on national developments or accepted good practice.

Monitoring the quality of care of a provider by the purchaser may be achieved through several approaches, including:

- monitoring the contract
- receiving regular reports on the provider's compliance with the Patient's Charter
- receiving reports on activity, waiting times, waiting lists, throughput and length of stay
- reports on complaints and litigation
- visiting the provider units and monitoring selected indicators of quality
- asking the general public about the quality of care and service received
- the setting-up of help lines.

The Dorset Health Commission's Approach

To give further insight into the process of monitoring quality, Denise Holden, on behalf of the Dorset Health Commission, has set out their approach and views on the need to develop such a process.

Figure 18

Developing the Commissioning Function of Health Authorities

Introduction: Setting the Context

'Working for Patients' created the purchaser/provider split as a central component of recent reforms. Initial focus was on the development of the provider function and the preparation for hospitals and community services to assume Trust status. The increasing impact of GP fundholders on service provision, although sporadically spread across the country, has also received considerable attention.

Developing the Purchasing Function

The term 'purchasing', as presently applied to Health Authorities, describes a series of activities that identifies the health and health service needs of individuals with a defined population. Those needs are then met through the purchase of a range of health services, both locally and nationally.

This process is underpinned by a range of values that influence the purchase and provision of health services and contracting cycle. Broadly these are based on the following:

- a clear focus on the delivery of high quality value for money health services
- commitment to delivery of public services, not necessarily from the public sector
- reward for performance
- promotion of patient choice
- increased individual and organisational accountability
- more efficient use of resources
- improved effectiveness
- continuous improvement in service access technical competence and consideration of patients and other service users as individuals.

Purchasing of health care is a relatively new function within the National Health Service. As such it is still evolving and Health Authorities are having to develop new skills and competencies to meet the responsibilities placed on them. This process of change will continue as DHAs and FHSAs merge to form Health Commissions with a still broader range of responsibilities spanning secondary and primary care. The agenda facing purchasers during coming years will be dominated by:

- maintenance and improvement of access times for inpatient and outpatient care. This must develop to include the reshaping of acute hospital settings as increases in primary care, changes in work practice and medical technology move forward rapidly;
- changes in service patterns that will flow from primary care being the principal focus for health;

➤

114

- increased GP fundholding and the development of GPs as providers of a wider range of community and potentially some acute services (e.g. private sector, GPs, voluntary organisations and nursing homes);
- a focus on health promotion and benefit balanced with a need to deliver high quality health services with ever increasing resource pressures;
- higher consumer expectations and a better informed public more willing to challenge professional models of care;
- increased expectations from the centre for the NHS to deliver the agenda locally;
- need for innovation and creative solutions in response to diminishing resources in order to ensure that the care provided is both effective and appropriate.

As implementation of the reforms has progressed so the need for greater clarity about the role and function of health care purchasers has emerged. This is in part driven by four considerations:

- the move to merge District Health Authorities and Family Health Service Authorities: although legislation is still awaited, many Authorities are establishing a joint approach to the provision of health services across primary, community and secondary care;
- the acknowledgement that Health Authorities were not simply purchasers or buyers of health care services but had responsibilities to local people to shape and direct the way in which the full range of health services were delivered within a defined area. The term 'Commission' acknowledges this broader remit although the extent to which this has been developed in local contexts varies across the country;
- increasingly Health Authorities are required to work collaboratively with a range of other agencies whose activities have an impact on the health status of individuals. Alliance with social services, education, housing and probation services are but a small example of the range of specific initiatives that have been established. Additionally Health Authorities are held accountable to the public they serve and are expected to increase the extent to which patients and the public influence the health services available;
- the emerging national framework provides the strategic context within which Health Authorities are required to work, allocation of resources and assessment of performance are judged on the basis of the progress with the delivery of the national agenda, including national policies such as Health of the Nation and Patient's Charter Rights and Standards.

The recent NHS Executive document 'Managing the New NHS: Functions and Responsibilities' provides a timely analysis of the functions that Health Authorities, and others within the NHS, will be

→

required to deliver. The principles underpinning the document are informed by the twin objectives of increasing the responsiveness of health services to local people and securing value for money for patients and the public from the resources spent on health care provision.

It is within this context that relationships between Health Authorities and health care providers will be shaped in the future. Before moving on to explore some of the specific characteristics likely to shape these relationships it is perhaps worth stating certain salient points that are likely to influence the development of health services in the future. These apply to Health Authorities and health care providers alike:

- funding will be driven by the ability to demonstrate health gain or benefit as well as the effective use of resources;
- need for greater clarity about the impact of care provided. Clinical practice must be up-dated in the light of the findings of research and development as well as feedback from individuals reviewing care (including, where appropriate, relatives and carers). Treatment or interventions that are not agreed to be effective will increasingly be excluded from contracts;
- traditional patterns of service delivery will be tested and challenged. If health care can be effectively provided in the primary or community care setting then that is where it will be made available.
- the commissioning function will focus increasingly on health gain. Provision of traditional health services is one of many ways to achieve this;
- private sector providers will be considered alongside public sector when awarding contracts;
- proxy measure of performance such as activity and through-put will be replaced by more sensitive measures of effectiveness and efficiency, based on delivery of anticipated health benefit to local people.

Moving forward with the agenda

The points highlighted above indicate the magnitude of change that is likely to characterise health services over the coming years. The oft-cited return to stability will not happen for either Health Authorities or service providers.

Anticipating that many of the points raised above will already be impacting on health care purchasers it is likely that the following will shape the work programmes of Health Authorities in the short to medium-term future.

- **evaluation of the health and health care needs of a defined population**

  This evaluation must be informed by a variety of sources including

→

demographic and research data, mortality and morbidity data, lifestyle factors, views of local people and the views of alliance partners. National and local input is essential to ensure that the evaluation is as robust as possible. Additionally the Health Authority must satisfy itself that the health needs assessment reflects the entire population, including hard to reach and less articulate groups.

- **establishing a local health strategy in response to local health needs that takes account of national priorities and policies** This strategy cannot be developed in isolation and should take account of the views of GPs (both fundholders and non-fundholders), local people, providers as well as other statutory and non-statutory agencies. The strategy should address resourcing implication and define clear priorities in the local context.

- **implementation of the health strategy** as the means by which resources are deployed to achieve delivery of priorities. Delivery is agreed through contracts for services placed with NHS and other providers. At present the main focus of many contracts is on maintaining and improving access times for inpatient and outpatient care, reshaping of acute services to increase day surgery provision, managing appropriate service shifts to primary or community care settings, improving clinical effectiveness and responding to advances in medical technology. As primary care becomes the principal focus for health, then changes in the pattern of service delivery becomes inevitable, requiring careful management by all concerned. Health Authorities will need to consider a range of options to achieve defined shifts, be clear about the benefits to be anticipated and take account of the impact of introducing new patterns of care and other service providers. In many areas primary care providers are able to extend the range of services available, in other circumstances 'outreach' services are provided by specialist centres with care delivered by community teams extended accordingly. This latter point is particularly relevant to the delivery of managed care, encouraging innovative joint working across a variety of different agencies be they public, private or voluntary.

Implementation of the strategy must also include mechanisms by which progress can be monitored and evaluated. At present this tends to concentrate on delivery of the contract requirements in terms of cost, activity and, less frequently, quality. Increasingly these proxy measures of performance will need to give way to a more sophisticated appraisal of the actual benefits delivered through investment in a particular service. Only by moving away from reliance on cost and activity measures will Health Authorities be in a position to demonstrate the actual changes in the health of the local population secured through delivery of strategic objectives. The development of clinical outcomes and effectiveness

➤

117

indicators in support of this objective is a highly complex area, that will nevertheless need to be addressed if Health Authorities and providers alike are to demonstrate how well they are performing.

- **building effective communications with local people** by seeking their views about health service delivery as well as providing feedback on the standards of care they should expect from health services. The Patient's Charter has served to raise people's expectations of health services and encourage them, quite rightly, to challenge providers when these expectations are not met. Furthermore local people must have an opportunity to influence the range and scope of health services purchased on their behalf, the values underpinning the health strategy, the focus of purchasing intentions and determination of priorities must all take account of the widely differing views of local people. Health Authorities cannot only represent the preferences of the most vocal or articulate.

  Hard-to-reach groups or those who may not normally be represented must be involved as fully as possible. It must also be remembered that local people are invaluable sources of intelligence regarding the actual case provided and means of improving delivery. Input into service reviews and development of contract specifications represent another key area on which Health Authorities must focus, and will increasingly be required to act on behalf of service users. Being responsive to local people is a complex process that cannot take place in a vacuum. Health Authorities must be prepared to invest in building relationships and networks with a wide range of different audiences. Not only funding but staff time and senior management commitment is necessary to succeed in achieving this area. It is not only service users and the general public that have a contribution to make. Carers, relatives, CHCs, voluntary organisations, local clinicians, GPs, GP fundholders, dentists, pharmacists and opticians as well as social, housing and education services are amongst the many who have a contribution to make. The key for Health Authorities is to ensure that the right audience is engaged in the right way at the right time.

- **a need to develop far more sophisticated and relevant sources of data regarding the performance of health services** There is little or no data available regarding the effectiveness of a range of clinical interventions and treatments. Data currently collected can only act as proxies to indicate a particular level of performance, often focusing attention on measures of process and input rather than results. Furthermore we are generally unable to track the way in which individuals move from one part of the service to another, the appropriateness of referral and use of diagnostic procedures. Application of the imperfect knowledge we do have can lead to

➤

perverse incentives and inappropriate use of resources providing
ineffective care. We must work jointly with providers, clinicians,
GPs and others to begin to develop more meaningful measures of
performance. This must also include a willingness by Health
Authorities to ask only for that data or information that is relevant.
Data for data's sake is also a waste of opportunity and resource.
By linking together meaningful data on clinical effectiveness with
feedback on performance from local people and other sources,
Health Authorities will find themselves increasingly well placed to
demonstrate the health benefits secured through the delivery of
their strategic objectives and work collaboratively with providers to
improve and enhance service delivery across all sectors.

Monitoring and Evaluation of Performance
The changes in the role and responsibility of Health Authorities
outlined above will necessitate accompanying changes in the means
by which performance is monitored and evaluated.

Present mechanisms rely primarily on process indicators of
performance that are focused on speed of access to services,
throughput of a particular service (normally measured in terms of
'finished consultant episodes') and overall cost. Quality standards and
criteria are often (but not always) included within contract
specifications. The reliance that can be placed on this data as
representing acceptable levels of performance by both purchaser and
provider is under intense scrutiny. The extent to which payment for
services should be linked for example to a finished consultant
episode does not address issues of appropriateness of referral or
effectiveness of treatment. Nor is there necessarily any evidence that
the patient derives any benefit from the care provided. Indeed in
some circumstances there may be a negative impact on the
individuals health.

At present monitoring arrangements are reliant on data from
providers that is generally retrospective in focus. The broad areas
covered with quality requirements tending to be built around:

- compliance with a range of standards;
- confirmation (via exception reporting) that a range of processes are
  in place. If there is a problem with a particular process providers
  are expected to report progress towards implementation;
- reporting back on clinical audit activity (but not necessarily action
  initiated);
- occasional 'quality visits' to ensure that contract requirements are
  being adhered to.

In addition to the above there are a plethora of national initiatives
aimed at measuring and monitoring. Accreditation, BS5750/ISO 9000
and the Royal College Guidelines are just three examples. Often
these are required in parallel to the quality specifications of different

➤

purchasers. In some instances this can result in a provider needing to respond to more than 60 different contract data requirements, creating an unwarranted demand that, it can be argued, has little relevance to the quality of experience of care for an individual nor the eventual outcome.

Monitoring that is based on these indicators alone is not an effective means of judging service delivery, additionally the extent to which it informs either purchaser or provider must be questioned. The tendency of the NHS to develop even more complex data for monitoring purposes must be addressed if the service is not to generate a bureaucracy based on inspection, regulation and policing. Each of these elements have their place. However this must be considered in the context of the scope for purchasers and providers to work collaboratively to eradicate waste and inefficiency whilst improving service quality.

The scene set by Denise Holden is one of continuous change led by the desire to improve both the service and care for patients. Monitoring of quality is clearly at several levels, as described in Chapter 1, with national bodies, purchasers and providers all working to ensure that patients and their families receive good quality care.

Everyone has a part to play in ensuring that patients receive the best possible quality of care within the available resources. I hope that the information within this book has given you more knowledge and helps to enable you to contribute, as part of the health care team, to the Quality Assurance initiatives in your particular hospital or Trust.

Exercise 6

- List the areas of a provider unit that should be monitored to ensure that patients are receiving good quality care.
- How often should the areas you have listed be
  — monitored
  — reported on
  — reviewed
  — visited?

References

1. *Operational principles* (EL(89)MB/169), (Department of Health)
2. Maxwell, in *British Medical Journal*, **288**, 12 May 1984: 1470–72.

Further Reading

Department of Health, *Working for Patients: Contracts for Health Services – Operational Principles.*

Morgan, J., M. Marchment and M. Russell, 'Introducing quality assurance to managers at unit level', *Hospital and Health Services Review*, April 1988, 65–9.

Glossary of Terms

Accreditation
'the process by which an Agency or Organisation evaluates and recognises a programme of study or institution as meeting predetermined Standards' (World Health Organisation, glossary of terms prepared for European Training Course on Quality Assurance, 1986)

Anticipated recovery pathway (ARP)
The anticipated pattern of recovery for a patient with a particular case-type or condition, the pathway includes all major interventions and events, in a planned sequence of time delivered by the multidisciplinary team. An ARP is a tool used to review the process of care delivery to patients.

Assessment
'the thorough study of a known or suspected problem in quality of care, designed to refine causes and necessary action to correct the problem' (World Health Organisation, glossary of terms prepared for European Training Course on Quality Assurance, 1986)

Care protocol/pathway
This is designed to be used as the record of care which through charting variance enables clinical audit to become part of the routine practice of care.

Clinical audit
A systematic, critical analysis of the quality of clinical care, which includes the procedures used for diagnosis and treatment, the use of resources and the resulting outcome for the patient.

Clinical pathway
A condensed flowchart (pathway) depicting key sequential events and expected progress through an episode of care. When a patient's progress diverts from the pathway for any reason it is documented as a variance, plus the reason for the deviance.

Clinical review
'The term clinical review is used to describe any evaluation activities which review the care being given to patients and the effectiveness of that care. Included in clinical review may be utilisation review activities.' (Australian Council on Hospital Standards, *Glossary of Terms*)

Concurrent audit (open chart audit)
Audit or examination of the patient or client's charts and records while the patient or client is still in hospital or being cared for at home, to establish if outcomes are being achieved for the patient or client

Concurrent review
Methods of assessing the quality of patient care while the patient is still in the hospital or being cared for – examples include: open chart audit or concurrent audit, patient interview or observation, staff interview or observation and group conferences.

Continuous quality improvement
'Consists, at a minimum, of three essential elements:

- efforts to know the customer ever more deeply and to link that knowledge ever more closely to day-to-day activities of the organisation
- efforts to mould the culture of the organisation, largely through the deeds of leaders, to foster pride, joy, collaboration and scientific thinking
- efforts to continuously increase knowledge of control over variation in the processes of work through widespread use of the scientific methods of collection, analysis and action upon data

When all these three efforts are developed in synchrony in an organisation, continuous improvement flourishes' (Donald M. Bewick).

Criterion

(i) 'variable selected as a relevant indicator of the quality of nursing care; a measure by which nursing care is judged as good' (B. W. Gallant and A. M. McLane, 'Outcome Criteria – a Process for Validation at Unit Level', *Journal of Nursing and Administration* [1979] **9**, 14–20)

(ii) 'statement which is measurable, reflecting the intent of a standard' (N. Lang, 'Issues in Quality Assurance in Nursing', *ANA Issues in Evaluative Research* [1976])

Critical path

A tool which identifies the key elements of patients' care which must occur within planned resources and activities for a specific diagnosis or procedure, and at the same time considers the time frames which must be followed to achieve the best possible patient outcome

Data collection

The collection of information concerning the topic to be researched or the patient. For example, data collection concerning a patient would include: information about his or her past and present health status and daily living pattern. This would include subjective data as described by the patient or his or her family, and objective data gleaned from observation and examination and documented data from records and reports.

Evidenced-based clinical practice

Practice based on recognised research evidence which is proven to be effective

Integrated care plan

Part of a clinical pathway which amalgamates into a written document all the elements of day-to-day care/treatment provided by the multidisciplinary team for each individual patient.

Evaluation
The process of determining the extent to which goals or objectives have been achieved

Monitoring
'the ongoing measurement of a variety of indicators of health care quality to identify problems' (World Health Organisation, glossary of terms prepared for European Training Course on Quality Assurance, 1986)

Nursing audit
A formal and detailed systematic review of nursing records in order to evaluate the quality of nursing care

Nursing care plan
A written statement of the patient or client's problems, expected outcomes and planned nursing interventions

Nursing history
A written record of information collected by a nurse when interviewing the patient, family or significant other

Nursing intervention
'specific nursing activities carried out by a nurse and on behalf of the patient' (Royal Australian Nursing Federation, 1985)

Nursing process
'the application of a problem-solving approach to nursing care. The four phases are:

- **assessment** – the collection and interpretation of data and the identification of patient problems
- **planning** – the determination of priorities, expected outcome and nursing interventions
- **implementation** – the delivery of planned nursing interventions
- **evaluation** – a continuous activity which compares actual outcomes with expected outcomes and which directs modifications of nursing care as required.'

Nursing standard
'a valid definition of the quality of nursing care that includes the criteria by which the effectiveness of care can be evaluated' (K. J. Mason, *How to Write Meaningful Nursing Standards*, 2nd edn (John Wiley & Sons, 1984)

Outcome criteria
Describes the desired effect of care in terms of patient behaviour responses, level of knowledge and health status

Outcome standards
'define the expected change in the client's health status and environment following nursing care and the extent of the client's satisfaction with nursing care' (K. J. Mason, *How to Write Meaningful Nursing Standards*, 2nd edn (John Wiley & Sons, 1984)

Patient questionnaire
Questionnaires developed to ask patients about care received, either in hospital or at home

Peer review
'evaluation of the quality of patient care by persons equivalent in status to those providing the care' (Australian Council on Hospital Standards, *Glossary of Terms*)

Philosophy
'a statement of a set of values and benefits which guide thoughts and actions' (Royal Australian Nursing Federation, 1985)

Process criteria
Relate to actions taken by nurses in order to achieve certain results and include: the assessment of techniques and procedures; the method of delivery of nursing care; interventions; techniques; how resources are used; the evaluation of care planned and given.

Protocols
A system of tracking either patient care or a service, and identifying and documenting the correct processes and activities within set time scales to an agreed outcome

Quality assurance

'the measurement of the actual level of the services rendered plus the efforts to modify, when necessary, the provision of these services in the light of the results of measurement' (World Health Organisation, glossary of terms prepared for European Training Course on Quality Assurance, 1986)

Quality control system

This is a system used in industry to check the quality of goods. In nursing it would refer to the quality of the environment and surroundings in which nurses work and patient care is given.

Quality of care

Degree of excellence

Quality planning

Involves four components:

- **Identifying** the customers of a particular process
- **Measuring** customer needs and expectations of the process and its outputs
- **Designing** a product or service responsive to their needs
- **Developing** the processes capable of producing the desired output.

Quality programme

'a documented set of activities, resources and events serving to implement the quality system of an organisation' (European Organisation for Quality Control, *Glossary of Terms used in the Management of Quality*, 5th edn, 1981)

Resource management

The balance of quality, cost and quantity

Retrospective audit (chart audit/closed audit)

Audit or examination of the patient or client's charts and records after he or she has been discharged to determine the quality of nursing care received

Retrospective review
Methods of assessing the quality of patient care after discharge, including retrospective chart audit; post-care interviews; post-care staff conferences; post-care questionnaires

Standard
(i) 'optimum level of care against which performance is compared' (B. W. Gallant and A. M. Mclane, 'Outcome Criteria – a Process for Validation at Unit Level', *Journal of Nursing and Administration* [1979] **9**, 14–20)

(ii) 'agreed upon level of excellence' (N. Lang, 'Issues in Quality Assurance in Nursing, *ANA Issues in Evaluation Research*, 1976)

Standard statements
Professionally agreed levels of performance appropriate to the population addressed which reflect what is acceptable, achievable, observable and measurable

Structure criteria
Items and services which enable the system to function and include the organisation of nursing services – recruitment, selection, manpower establishments and skill mix; equipment; ancillary services – such as supplies, central sterilising, catering, pharmacy, laboratory services, laundry, paramedical services and the provision of buildings; agreed rules and regulations, policies and procedures.

Total quality management
'is the system by which quality at each interface is ensured. It is an approach to improving the effectiveness and flexibility of the service as a whole – a way of organising and involving the whole service, every Authority, unit, department, activity, every single person at every level to ensure that organised activities happen the way they are planned, and seeking continuous improvement in performance.' (B. Morris, 'Total Quality Management', *International Journal of Health Care Quality Assurance* [1989] 2(3), 4–6)

Index

Abdellah, F.   2, 25
Abraham, S. C. S.   94
accreditation   5, 15, 16, 119
Ager, J. W.   25
Alcott, L. M.   1, 25
Area Health Authorities   3
audit
  clinical   12, 18–19, 33, 119;
    accident reports and 85;
    action plan after 88;
    analysis of 87; areas for
    82–3, 91; benefits of 73–4;
    care plans and 85; change
    as result of 78, 79, 87–8;
    commitment to 81, 90;
    communication and 78–9,
    89, 90; Complaints Reports
    and 85; confidentiality and
    79–80, 86, 90; criteria for
    85, 91–2; cycle 71–3; data
    for 85–6, 87, 90; definition
    of 71; evidence base for 84;
    forms for 86; improvements
    after 87; indicators for 85,
    87, 92–3; interviews in 86;
    management and 79, 81, 82,
    83; mission statements and
    75; need for 73; objectives
    of 75, 79, 80, 84, 90;
    outcomes of 80, 87–8, 89,
    90; patients and 73, 78, 86,
    92–3; philosophy of care
    and 75; principles of 74–9;
    problems of 79–81; quality
    assurance strategy and 82;
    questionnaires in 86;
    reasons for 79; research and
    84; resources for 79, 81, 83,
    90; results of 80, 87–8, 89,
    90; scope of 82–3, 84, 90;
    size of 80, 87, 90; staff
    involvement in 73, 79–81,
    83–4, 89, 90; standards and
    75–8, 80, 85; success of
    81–8, 89–90; time for 84, 90
  concurrent   22
  cycle. change, appropriate
    72–3; current practice 71;
    expectations/reality of 72;
    standards, setting of in 72
  local   14, 15
  medical   5, 11–13, 33
  national   14–15
  nursing   12, 17–18
  open-chart   22
  retrospective   22
  standards: monitoring of,
    comparison with 68,
    75–6; principles of in 77–8
  see also King's Fund
    Organisational Audit;
    quality assurance;
    standards
Audit Commission   13, 14–15,
  17, 46
Australia, health care standards
  in   5, 15, 17, 19

Baker, A.   26
Baker, F.   109
Ball, J.   6, 9, 26
Balme, H.   2, 25

Index

Index

monitoring of by
  purchasers 111–121
standards for 45, 46–7
see also audit; care; markets,
  care and
purchasers
  agenda for 114–16
  contracts, quality assurance
    and 17, 18, 117, 118–19
  function of 115
  monitoring of providers
    by 111–121
  purchasing function,
    development of 114–16
  role of 115
  standards for 45, 46–7
  see also markets, care and

quality, dimensions of 111
quality assurance
  audit and 82
  background to 1 5, 10
  communications and 3, 30,
    32, 118
  contracts and 17, 18, 111–13,
    118–9
  cost effectiveness of 1
  criteria for 20–1
  cycle of 43–4
  definition of 13, 39
  evaluation: levels of 16–18;
    sources for 116–17; 118–19;
    structures for 3, 5, 19–25, 33
  funding and 5
  General Managers and 10
  Griffiths Report and 4
  health strategies and 117–18
  indicators for 48, 90,
    117–18, 119, 120
  measurement of 21–3, 30, 31,
    33, 39, 116
  monitoring and 13–15, 33,
    119–20; Dorset Health
    Commission 113–20
  objectives of 20
  Ombudsman and 4
  patients' attitudes and 2–3,
    5–9, 22, 29

programme (QAP) 19, 20
research into 4–5, 20–1
responsibility for 10
standards in *see* standards
systems for: Monitor 6–9;
  Rush Medicus 5–6
TQM and 29–35
training for 30
WHO and 12
see also audit

Quality Patient Care Scale 4

Redfern, S. 94
Regional Health Authorities 46
Reiter, F. 3, 25
Roberts, C. J. 26
Royal College of General
  Practitioners 11, 12, 17, 18
Royal College of Nursing
  Standards of Care
    Project 10, 40–2
  Standards of Nursing Care 41,
    68, 119
  Towards Standards 41–2, 68
Royal College of
  Physicians 12, 17, 18, 94
Royal College of Surgeons 12,
  17, 18
Royal Commission on the
  National Health Service
  (Morrison) 4, 12
Rush Medicus 5–6
Russell, M. 121

St James' Hospital, Leeds,
  clinical protocol 95–106
Sale, D. N. T. 69
Salmon Report 3
Schmadl, J. C. 13, 26
Shaw, C. 94
Slater Nursing Competencies
  Rating Scale 4
staff
  accountability of 41–2
  audits and 73, 79–81, 83–4, 90
  individual commitment
    of 33

135

Index

TQM and 32, 33–34, 35; *see
also* quality assurance and
universal 45, 46
USA 1, 2, 3, 4, 5–6, 13, 15
use of 42
writing of 37–8, 44–5,
47–56, 63–9
Stewart, I. 1, 25
Standards 1–2
Stewart, S. D. 25

teams, multidisciplinary
audits by 12–13, 73, 74–5,
79, 83, 91–3
care by 18–19; philosophy of
75
clinical protocols and 106,
107, 108
evaluation by 2
group conferences and 22
standards and 47–8, 63–4, 77
TQM and 30, 32, 33
Total Quality Management
(TQM)
approach to 34
background to 29–31
concepts of 31–3

definition of 30
health care and 34, 35
NHS and 29–30, 32–4
patient care and 29–31,
32–4, 35
philosophy of 29
processes of 31–2
training, standards of 4, 30
see also staff

USA, health care standards
in 1, 2, 3, 4, 5–6, 13, 15,
16, 19

Walshe, K. 94
Wandelt, M. A. 25
Ward, M. J. 60, 68
Weiss, R. 109
Whelan, J. 27
Whitehead, A. G. W. 26
Whitehead, T. 26
Williamson, J. D. 26
Williamson, J. W. 13, 26
Working for Patients 12

Zander, K. 109
Zell, D. 109